Manual Medicine 1984

Results of the International Seminar Week in Fischingen, Switzerland

Edited by
J. Dvořák, V. Dvořák, and W. Schneider

Methodic-didactic Consultants:
E. Schegg and T. Tritschler

Translated by
W. G. Gilliar

With 296 Figures

Springer-Verlag
Berlin Heidelberg New York Tokyo

Jiri Dvořák, M.D.
Department of Neurology, University of Bern
Inselspital, 3010 Bern, Switzerland

Vaclav Dvořák, M.D.
Bahnhofstraße 10, 7402 Bonaduz, Switzerland

Werner Schneider, M.D.
Hauptstraße 39, 8280 Kreuzlingen, Switzerland

Methodic-didactic Consultants:

Ernst Schegg, Ph.D., Educational Center of the SBG (Swiss Bank Union)
Wolfsberg, 8272 Ermatingen, Switzerland

Thomas Tritschler, Director of the school for Physiotherapy, Kantonsspital
8208 Schaffhausen, Switzerland

Translator:

Wolfgang G. Gilliar, Michigan State University, College of Osteopathic Medicine, A319 E. Fee Hall, East Lansing, MI 48824-1316, USA

The figure on the cover is identical to figure 5 in the book.
Colored symbols are explained there.

ISBN-13: 978-3-642-70219-8 e-ISBN-13: 978-3-642-70217-4
DOI: 10.1007/978-3-642-70217-4

Library of Congress Cataloging in Publication Data. Manuelle Medizin 1984. English. Manual medicine 1984. Papers presented at an international seminar during the week following the 7th International Congress of the International Federation of Manual Medicine, held Sept. 1983, in Zurich, sponsored by the Swiss Federation of Manual Medicine. Translation of: Manuelle Medizin 1984. 1. Manipulation (Therapeutics)-Congresses. I. Dvořák, J. (Jiri), 1948- . II. Dvořák, V. (Vaclav), 1945- . III. Schneider, W. (Werner), 1941- . IV. International Federation of Manual Medicine. International Congress (7th : 1983 : Zurich, Switzerland) V. Schweizerische Ärztegesellschaft für Manuelle Medizin. VI. Title. [DNLM: 1. Manipulation, Orthopedic-congresses. 2. Physical Medicine-congresses. WB 460 M294m 1983 a]
RM724.M3513 1985 615.8'2 85-2789

Typesetting, Offsetprinting and Binding: Appl, 8853 Wemding, Germany
2119/3140-5 4 3 2 1 0

Preface

Commissioned by the Swiss Federation of Manual Medicine and under the patronage of FIMM (International Federation of Manual Medicine) we conducted an international seminar during the week following the 7th International Congress of FIMM (Zuerich/Switzerland - September 1983).
Thirty Manual Medicine experts had come together in the education center of the Cloister Fischingen secluded in the eastern part of Switzerland and away from any city life, to discuss in a week long seminar the status of Manual Medicine.

Working together in the form of several groups, the following points were emphasized:
- terminology
- diagnostic criteria (are Manual Medicine findings reproducible?)
- therapeutic interventions (degree of congruity of treatment plans)

The participants demonstrated great enthusiasm and commitment, and so it was possible to have the content of the individual group's discussion communicated to and presented for further scrutiny to all participants during the seminar week.
As members of the organizing committee and as the editors of this publication, we hope to help establish a more standardized international terminology concerning the field of Manual Medicine.
As this clinical trial (investigating the diagnostic reliability and the therapeutic efficiency of MM) shows, factors such as terminology, diagnostic criteria and therapeutic plans are a prerequisite for multi-center studies.
Only when the language is a comprehensible one and when the methods used in Manual Medicine have been completely scrutinized by members of this field, will Manual Medicine be able to present its knowledge to members of traditional medicine and finally gain general acceptance.
The participants of the Fischingen Seminar Week were aware of this fact and agreed that one has to work towards that goal.
We are pleased and very grateful that the Springer Verlag was willing to publish this publication and to present the results obtained during the week's sessions in such a clear and organized manner. We hope to hereby make available to all interested colleagues the status of Manual Medicine in 1983/84. We would want to hope that the reproducibility of the various diagnostic procedures and the success of the therapeutic intervention will be further evaluated and communicated in the national chapters of FIMM. Only then will one be able to determine the final success of the Seminar Week in Fischingen.
The editors want to thank the Swiss Federation of Manual Medicine for its active and financial support of this seminar week. Special thanks are extended to Dr. H. D. Neumann who constantly encouraged us with his practical advice.
We want to further thank Mr. Muehlemann, director of the Swiss Union Bank, and Dr. E. Schegg, also of the Swiss Union Bank (the Education Center, Wolfsberg) for their support and advice. The group-dynamics assistance provided by Dr. Schegg greatly contributed to the success of this week.

We want to thank the secretaries, Ms. Maeder, Mrs. Grange and Mrs. B. Dvorak who during that week successfully deciphered the partially illegible manuscripts which had originally been brought forth in 7 languages. Special thanks go to Ms. Reichert who in record speed completed the final draft of the manuscript.
Due to technical reasons and time restrictions, we were not able to have all 30 contributors help in the task of proofreading of this work. The editors would herewith like to apologize for any possible errors and thank the critical reader for his/her understanding.

Note on Abbreviations

To ensure easy identification, the following abbreviations have been used in referring to countries:

A	Austria
AUS	Australia
CZE	Czechoslovakia
DEN	Denmark
F	France
FIN	Finland
FRG	Federal Republic of Germany
I	Italy
SWE	Sweden
SWI	Switzerland
UK	United Kingdom
USA	United States

Editor's Introduction

The authors of this book were the leaders of the organizing committee which prepared the International Seminar Week under the sponsorship of the Swiss Federation of Manual Medicine and under the patronage of FIMM (International Federation of Manual Medicine). This book is the product of countless hours of conference prelanning, time during the seminar week, and in debriefing the results and placing them in this format.

The authors recognize the need for better definition and description of the terminology, diagnostic criteria, and therapeutic interventions utilized in the field of manual medicine. Literature in the field is published a number of languages and the terminology in the field is sufficiently confusing that translation presents great difficulty.

This attempt at addressing the problem was a monumental first step. Including members of the leadership of manual medicine worldwide representing twelve countries, teachers of eight different schools, and speaking seven different languages, was an innovative and most successful undertaking.

This English edition is an attempt to translate as accurately as possible not only the language but the meaning of the original German text. This book makes a valuable contribution to the literature in the field of manual medicine and can well serve as the basis for future effort towards standardization of language in the field and as a basis for study and clinical trials in the future.

Philip E. Greenman, D.O.
Wolfgang Gilliar, B.S.

Table of Contents

List of Contributors

Alder Jean, M. D., leitender Arzt, Orthopädische Universitätsklinik, Balgrist, Forchstraße 340, 8008 Zurich, Switzerland

Allen Thomas, D. O., Professor, Dean, Chicago College of Osteopathic Med., 5200, Ellis Avenue, Chicago, IL 20615, USA

Baumgartner Hubert, M. D., Chief, Klinik Wilhelm Schulthess, Neumuensterallee 10, 8008 Zurich, Switzerland

Berger Meinhard, M. D., Department of Neurology of the University, 6020 Innsbruck, Austria

Beal Myron, D. O., Professor, College of Osteopathic Med., Michigan State University, 201 West Fee Hall, East Lansing, MI 48824, USA

Brugnoni Guido, M. D., Ospedale civile, 21049 Taradate, Italy

Burn Loic, M. D., The Stables, Upper Ham. Rd. Ham Common, Richtmond, United Kingdom

Fossgreen Johannes, M. D., Chief, Dept. of Rheumatology, Aarhus Amtssygehus University Hospital, 8000 Aarhus, Denmark

Geiger Rolf, M. D., Onkenstraße 19, 7600 Offenburg, W. Germany

Greenman Philip, D. O., Associate Dean, College of Osteopathic Med., Michigan State University, 309 East Fee Hall, East Lansing, MI 48824, USA

Gourjon Alain, M. D., 42, rue Paul Vlery, 75116 Paris, France

Haldemann Scott, M. D., D. C., 1125 East 17 St. Suite W117, Santa Ana, CA 91701, USA

Hamberg Jern, M. D., Chief, Box 94, 82200 Alfta, Sweden

Janda Vladimir, M. D., Professor, University Hospital, Srobarova 50, 10034 Prag 10, Czechoslovakia

Juvin Patrick, M. D., 42, rue Paul Valery, 75116 Paris, France

Kappler Robert, D. O., Professor, Chicago College of Osteopathic Med., 5200 Sellis Avenue, Chicago, IL 60615, USA

Kimberly Paul, D. O., Professor, 8377 17th Street N., St. Petersburg, FL 33702, USA

Lewit Karel, M. D., Central Railwy Health Inst., Italska 37, 25229 Dobrichovice 360, Czechoslovakia

Mildenberger Franz, M. D., Avagen 14, 78041 Gagnef, Sweden

Mohrle Alfred, M. D., Königsteiner Straße 68, 6232 Bad Soden/TS 1, W. Germany

Neumann Heinz-Dieter, M. D., Buhlertalstraße 45, 7580 Buhl, W. Germany

Paterson John K., M. D., Wimpole Street 14, London WIM 7 AB, United Kingdom

Rekola Kaj, M. D., Central hospital, Katajatie 11, 40250 Jyvaeskylae, Finland

Reynolds Herbert, Ph. D., Professor, College of Osteopathic Med., Michigan State University, East Lansing, MI 48824, USA

Seifert Klaus, M. D., Professor, Grosflecken 72, 2350 Neumunster, W. Germany

Schonenberger Felix, M. D., Belbergstraße 3, 3123 Belp/Bern, Switzerland

Schwarz Erich, M. D., Ca'da Nona, 6986 Novaggio, Switzerland

Trost Harry, M. D., Steinwiesstr. 4, 8032 Zurich, Switzerland

Waller Urs, M. D., Ernst Schulerstraße 5, 2502 Biel, Switzerland

Winer Conrad, E. R., LL. B., M. B., B. S., M. R. C. S., L. R. C. P., D. R. C. O. G., M. L. C. O. M., D. P. R. M., F. A. C. R. M., Osteopathic Physician. Director, Department of Physical Medicine & Rehabilitation, Royal Prince Alfred Hospital, Sydney, Australia.

Wolff Hanns-Dieter, M. D., Gartenfeldstraße 6, 5500 Trier, W. Germany

Chapter 1

Group Approach and Didactic Considerations

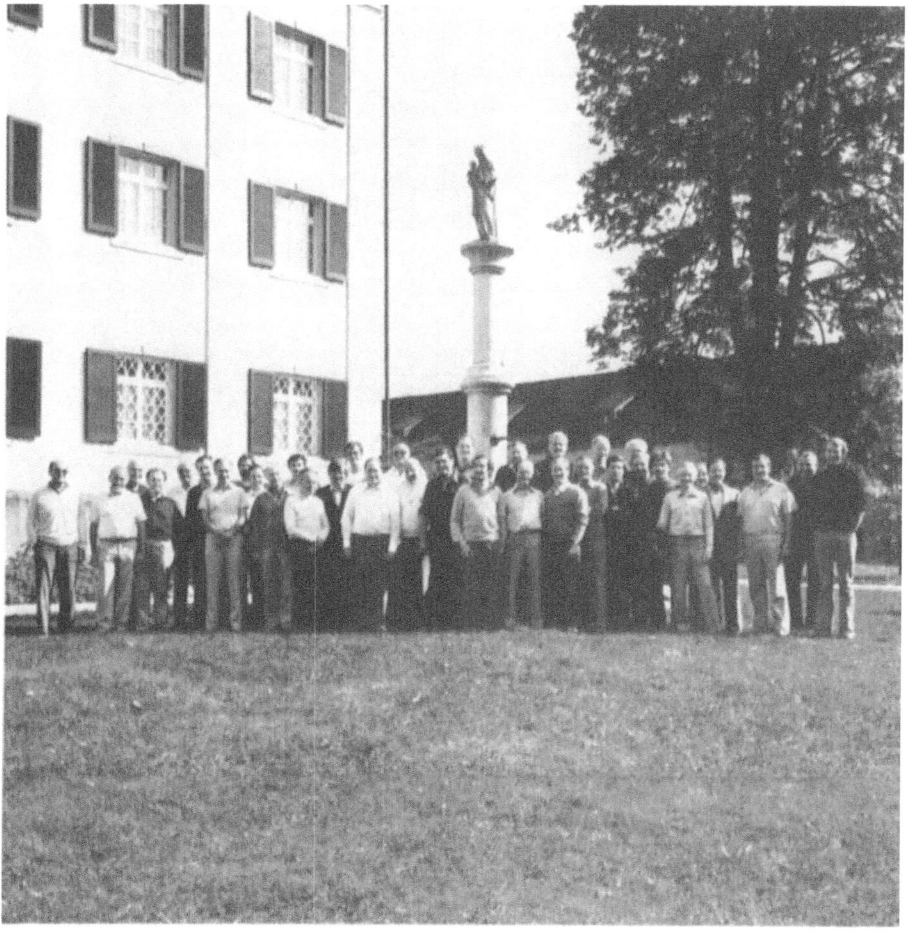

It seems that in today's world of ever increasing complexities Schiller's words "the strong are most powerful alone" has lost some of its validity. Thus, the compilation of a body of knowledge and of those manual medicine techniques used throughout the world is a task that – undoubtedly – can only be mastered by bringing together selected specialists in one group. The international seminar provided such a classical meeting, in which only through group effort would it be possible to approach different complex problems. As has been shown in other instances, group effort is far superior to individual solutions. Multidimensional aspects could then be approached more efficiently by the international group of experts.

To this effect, the Fishingen International Seminar Week of Manual Medicine was initiated, and organization and programming of the this week long meeting was directed towards dynamic group interaction. The following aspects were of importance when organizing the meeting:

- programming,
- time restrictions for individual work sessions,
- participant selection,
- group composition.

The timing of the program was arranged such that in the plenary session the information and ideas collected from the four sub-groups could be passed on to all participants. Following the individual groups' sessions were scheduled the general plenary meetings to provide insight to the overall progress. This challenged the groups to limit their discussions to a set time frame and provided them furthermore with specific goals. The general plenary sessions were found to be a quite useful and effective means of communication. Due to this schedule, the results could easily be formulated and kept up to date.

Of crucial importance is the specific goal that is associated with each group meeting, since this determines the quality of the task to be mastered. Each participant was provided with a written statement clearly defining the goal. It is thus the duty of the organizing personnel to assure that the goals are clear and unambiguous to every participant. By doing so, however, attention is to be paid not to provide undue discussion content preliminarily. The organizing personnel should limit their influence to the objective and didactic component of these proceedings.

Group composition arrangement, a task that requires significant and delicate preparation, should only be undertaken by the course chairpersons, since the success of the seminar is intricately connected with this process. It would not be correct to help establish so-called "ego clubs" in which the participants share the same opinions a priori.

In Fischingen, the diversity of the group's composition can be discerned by the different personalities, schools and countries. The language barriers resulting from this diversity were soon overcome by good will and enthusiasm. By the end of the week the differences in age, social status, country (12 countries and 7 different languages) were overshadowed by the quality of the work.

While physicians are known to be individualists, this seminar week in Fischingen served a greater purpose. Impressive were the willingness and enthusiasm with which the representatives participated as to actively and constructively cope with a great volume of work. Different opinions and critical issues were always treated with respect, which meant that at the end of the week the differences and similarities were articulated objectively without the intention to press for agreement. The overall working atmosphere was influenced by the time constraints put upon the individual groups, yet the chal-

lenge to define clearly the basic principles and help in one's understanding of them was successfully dealt with, all of which may have contributed – in retrospect – to the overall success of the real group effort.
Having limited a group to eight participants and with clear structural guidelines provided by the coordinating personnel made the dynamic group effort a successful one.

Program for the Group Sessions

1. Group Formation

- Chairman
- Secretary
- Informant
- Time assessor

2. Time Scheduling

3. Goal Formulation
- Content
- Documents needed
- Equipment/Aids

4. Group Work

5. General Meeting and Compilation of All Group Work Results

The final presentation was conducted in a similar fashion. This assured a clear and organized comminication of all of the groups' results.

Recommendation for Presentation

Goals:	General information for all participants and definition of the status of manual medicine in 1983.
Time Frame:	Total time allotted – 90 minutes: 10 minutes – general presentation 5 minutes – translations (summaries) 30 minutes – presentation of 10 specific diagnostic and therapeutic procedures 45 minutes – discussion.
Organization:	– Speaker for general topics – Summary speakers – Authors of 10 cases – Moderator – Time assessor.

This seminar week, in which 32 physicians participated – of whom a great number are university professors and have extensive didactic experience – demonstrated that with good organization, clear goals and instructions the efficiency of group sessions can be significantly improved leading to greater success, both personally and time wise.

It was a great experience to see a heterogenous group as this demonstrate such willingness to learn and to generally accept the meeting's organization and group dynamics. An accomplishment to which the beautiful surroundings and atmosphere of the the Cloister Fischingen probably contributed.

Terminology

An attempt has been made to standardize the language used in the different societies for manual medicine. In particular, the terms "manipulation" and "mobilization" needed further clarification, since, even though used in the different countries, they do have different meanings as to the type of treatment intervention they encompass in the individual country.

Manipulation

In the USA, manipulation refers to any therapeutic procedure in which the hands are used to treat the patient (thus a rather general term).
In Europe, manipulation refers to what is described in the English language or according to American osteopathic terminology as "high velocity, low amplitude thrust."

Mobilization

"Mobilization" is described in the USA as soft tissue and articulatory type of treatment (muscle energy technique), whereas in Europe this term refers to articular mobilization without thrusting force.

Thrust-Impulse Techniques

Both these terms describe the same entity, with "thrust" being preferred in the English language and "impulse" being more common in the European schools.
In this text, the terms "mobilization with impulse" and "mobilization without impulse" were chosen, and the individual treatment techniques are described as manipulative or mobilizing procedures, respectively.

Chapter 2

Controlled Patient Examination Trial

On September 12, 1983, twelve physicians from seven countries participated in a controlled patient examination trial. Six groups were formed with five of them being comprised of two physicians from the same country while the sixth group consisted of two physicians from two different countries (Czechoslovakia and Austria) since they can be considered to be representatives of the same school.

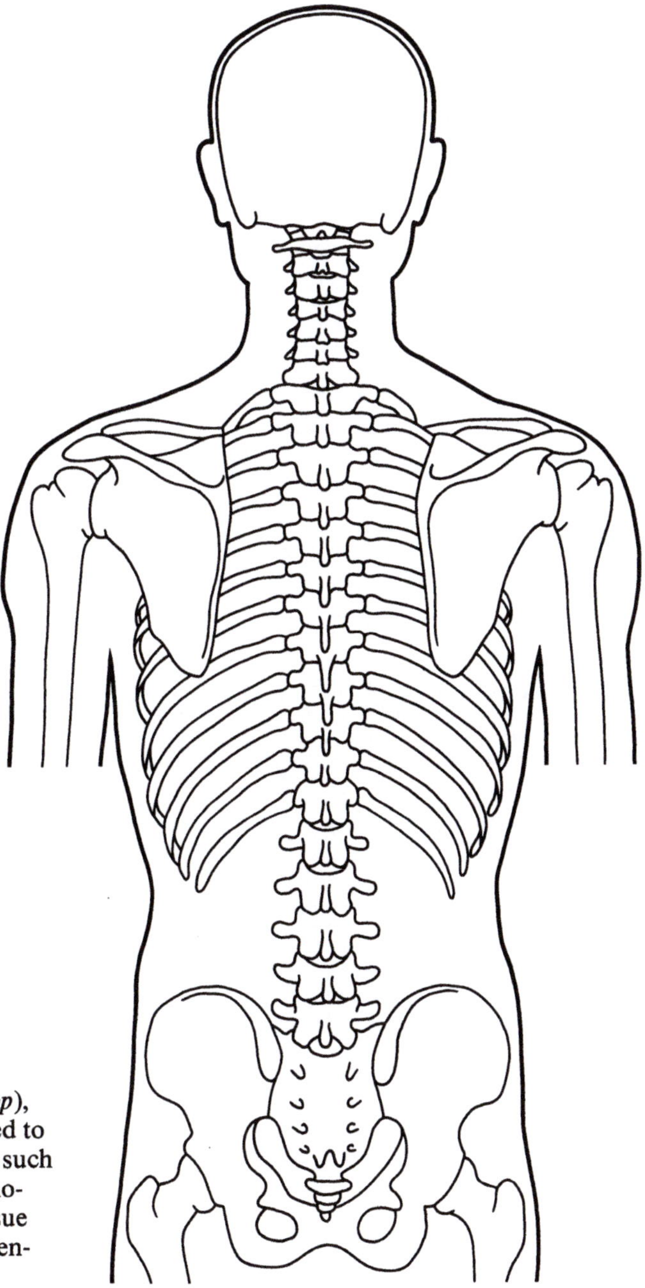

Fig. 1. Using the key (*top*), the examiners were asked to indicate on the diagram such diagnostic findings as motion restrictions, soft tissue abnormalities and myotendinosis

2.1 Can Manual Medicine Findings Be Reproduced?

(Results of a Small Controlled Clinical Trial)

Objective

To determine the extent of
- agreement among the representatives from the seven countries in regard to diagnostic manual-medicine findings
- agreement in regard to the congruity of the therapeutic approach.

Methods

Six typical cases dealing with musculo-skeletal problems were selected by a rheumatologist experienced in manual medicine.
Six pairs of physicians representing a total of seven countries (USA, United Kingdom, West Germany, Czechoslovakia, Austria, Switzerland and France) received a standardized 3-page protocol (Dvorak and Schneider, unpublished). On the first two pages of this protocol the functional and palpatory findings were recorded, while the third page was reserved for the recommendation of a therapeutic plan.
First, each pair of physicians examined one patient for minutes. The examiners received information about the patient's chief complaint but were not porvided with the complete past history at this stage. The examiners had been instructed to seek no further historical data from the patient (the patients had been instructed accordingly).
In the first 20 minutes, the examiners conducted their routine manual medicine examination, followed by a basic neurological and orthopedic examination. The examiners then recorded with non-erasable pen the major functional, pathological and palpatory findings on the accompanying examination forms. The three findings considered to be most significant were indicated by a circle (see examination protocol, pp. 10, 11).
The examiners' findings were then collected by a control person assigned to each individual group. Immediately a copy was made and stored in a different room. At this point the records of the first examination were redistributed to their respective groups, now along with a detailed past medical history and the results of previous laboratory results and radiological findings including the original X-rays. The examiners also obtained information about previous and present therapeutic interventions and the success thereof.
The group was allotted an additional 20 minutes for further patient examination and the preparation of a therapeutic plan.
The appropriate therapeutic plan was then recorded on the third page of the protocol, and the primary treatment modality was indicated by a circle by the individual examiner (Tables 1–6).
After spending a total of about 40 minutes with the patient, the examiners turned in these examination records to the control person; these records were then stored in sealed envelopes.
In the morning period, each group examined three different patients, and in the afternoon three additional patients were seen by each group.
The original examination protocol and its copies were stored in sealed envelopes.

Examination protocol: International Seminar Week, 9-12-1983

Examiner: ____________________ Patient: ____________________

1. Findings
1.1 Functional abnormalities at the axial skeleton

Area:

Spinal segment (indicated by .)

	L	R
C0–C3	☐	☐
C4–C6	☐	☐
C7–T3	☐	☐
T4–T8	☐	☐
T9–L2	☐	☐
L3–L5	☐	☐
L5–SIJ	☐	☐

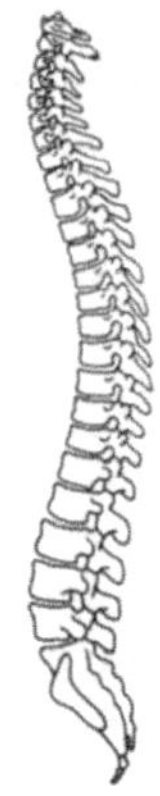

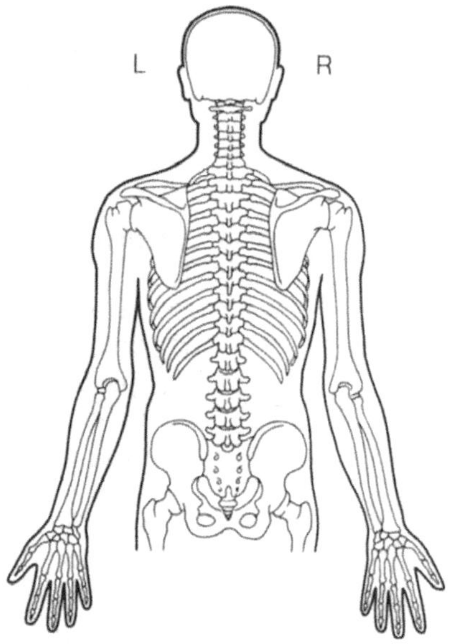

Classification of functional abnormality:

Area/Segment (according to 1.1)	☐	☐	☐	☐	☐
Hypomobility	☐☐	☐☐	☐☐	☐☐	☐☐
Hypermobility	☐☐	☐☐	☐☐	☐☐	☐☐
Positional asymmetry	☐☐	☐☐	☐☐	☐☐	☐☐

Remarks:

Examination protocol: International Seminar Week, 9-12-1983

Examiner: ______________________ Patient: ______________________

1.1 Palpatory findings at the axial skeleton

Spinal segment

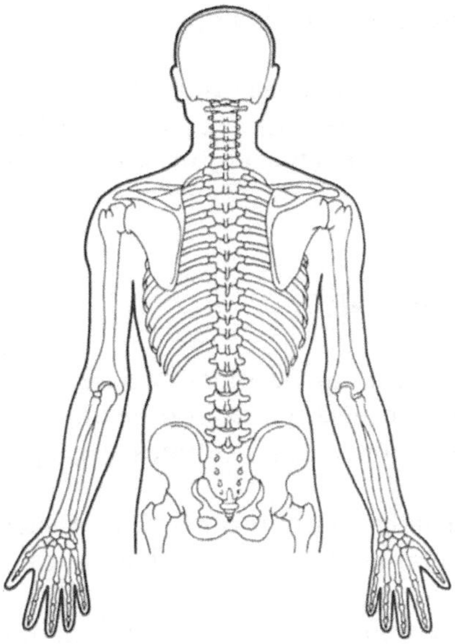

Area:	L	R	Skin-Subcutaneous Tissue	Muscles	Bone-Joints
C0–C3	☐	☐	☐	☐ ☐	☐ ☐
C4–C6	☐	☐	☐	☐ ☐	☐ ☐
C7–T3	☐	☐	☐	☐ ☐	☐ ☐
T4–T8	☐	☐	☐	☐ ☐	☐ ☐
T9–L2	☐	☐	☐	☐ ☐	☐ ☐
L3–L5	☐	☐	☐	☐ ☐	☐ ☐
L5–SIJ	☐	☐	☐	☐ ☐	☐ ☐

1.3 Functional Muscle Examination

	Shortened	Weakened	Other
Suboccipital muscles			
Trapezius muscle descending portion			
Levator scapulae muscle			
Semispinatus capitis muscle			
Sterocleidomastoid muscle			
Scalene muscles			
Rhomboid muscle			
Erector Spinae thoracis muscles			
Serratus anterior muscle			
Pectoralis anterior muscle			
Erector spinae lumborum muscles			
Abdominal muscles			
Iliopsoas muscle			
Gluteal muscles			
Piriformis muscle			
Rectus femoris muscle			
Adductor muscles			
Hamstring muscles			
Tensor fascia latae muscle			

Indicate the <u>three</u> most significant findings with ☒

To assure the validity of this trial, particular attention was paid that the physicians participating in the study would have no opportunity to communicate with each other nor to obtain further information about the individual patient.

2.2 Findings and Results (Diagnosis and Therapy)

Following is listed the information regarding the patient's chief complaint, relevant historical data and questions presented to the individual patient. The major findings from the respective groups are presented here in a similar fashion.

Patient 1: K.J., 32 Year Old Male

Chief Complaint: Following a car accident two years ago the patient had been suffering from repeated neck pains and headaches. Other complaints consist of not being able to concentrate at times and significant fatigue.[1]

Social History: The patient is married and owns a successful metal work shop. He performs both manual labor and office duties.

The insurance claims concerning the car accident had not been settled at the time of this examination, since the opinions of the physicians consulted in this case had not come to an agreement.

History of Chief Complaint: The patient was run over in a car accident two years ago. The patient indicated that he was unconscious for two hours. In the neurological unit of a Swiss Canton hospital, the diagnosis of a light concussion of the brain with post-traumatic syndrome was issued. An examination six months after the accident indicated normal neurostatus, but the patient complained of difficulties in concentration, blockage of thought processes, diminished physical fitness and headaches. The attending physician diagnosed a chronic, vasomotor myogenic tension-headache, recurrent disturbances in consciousness of undetermined origin and a general depressive status.
After one year and having worn a shoulder and head cast for several weeks, the patient reported some improvement of the previous complaints. Following the shoulder and head cast, the patient had worn a removable collar for several months. The patient had been using tranquilizers for a period of one year.

Laboratory Findings: Unremarkable.

X-ray Studies: X-rays were taken in the A–P and lateral projections, including maximal flexion and extension positions. The bony structures appeared intact and the intervertebral spaces normal. A significant increase in mobility was found in the segment of C4–C5.

1 This was the only information the examiners were provided with for their initial functional and palpatory examination

Problem: To what extent are the headaches and lack of concentration related to or the result of a post-traumatic syndrome? To what extent can the headaches be ascribed to spondylogenic problems?

Examination Findings (Fig. 2): As indicated by all six groups the bilateral hypomobility seen in the upper cervical spine (cranio-cervical junction) is the major finding. The hypomobility was assessed both functionally and by palpation with soft tissue evaluation (segmental zones of irritation).
Each group reported findings of increased tension, changes in homogeneity and painfulness in the sub-occipital musculature. Secondary findings, e.g., segmental dysfunctions in the cervico-thoracic junction (CZE, A, UK) and the sacroiliac joint (SWI, FRG) were indicated.
It is interesting to note that no other findings were reported (Figure 1).

Treatment Plan (Table 1): All groups, except the Czechoslovakian-Austrian group, thought that manipulation (impulse (thrust) techniques) at the cranio-cervical junction is contraindicated. The assessment of such a contraindication can be considered as quite significant.
The Swiss, Czechoslovakian and Austrian schools recommended soft-tissue mobilization, muscle energy techniques, and a soft cervical collar. The British school in addition recommends local anesthetic infiltration into the sub-occipital region.
The representatives from Germany and Switzerland would include manipulative treatment to the cervico-thoracic junction and the sacroiliac joints.

Authors' Remarks: The various complaints presented by patients suffering from trauma to the upper cervical spine or concussion of the brain often lead to controversial discussions among the consulting physicians. These multifarious viewpoints concerning some such complex problems are often reflected by the variability in expert opinions.
The authors deliberately chose this patient in order to confront the examining physicians with just this problem complex. It is noteworthy to realize that there was general agreement in regard to the functional and palpatory examinations of the vertebral column. Of further importance is the fact that there was agreement on therapeutic procedures especially those that were considered to be contraindicated (e.g. manipulation to the upper cervical spine). Classic manipulation to the cervical spine, however, should be differentiated from the soft tissue techniques, or the muscle energy techniques.

Fig. 2. Patient 1: K. J., 32 year old male; major findings

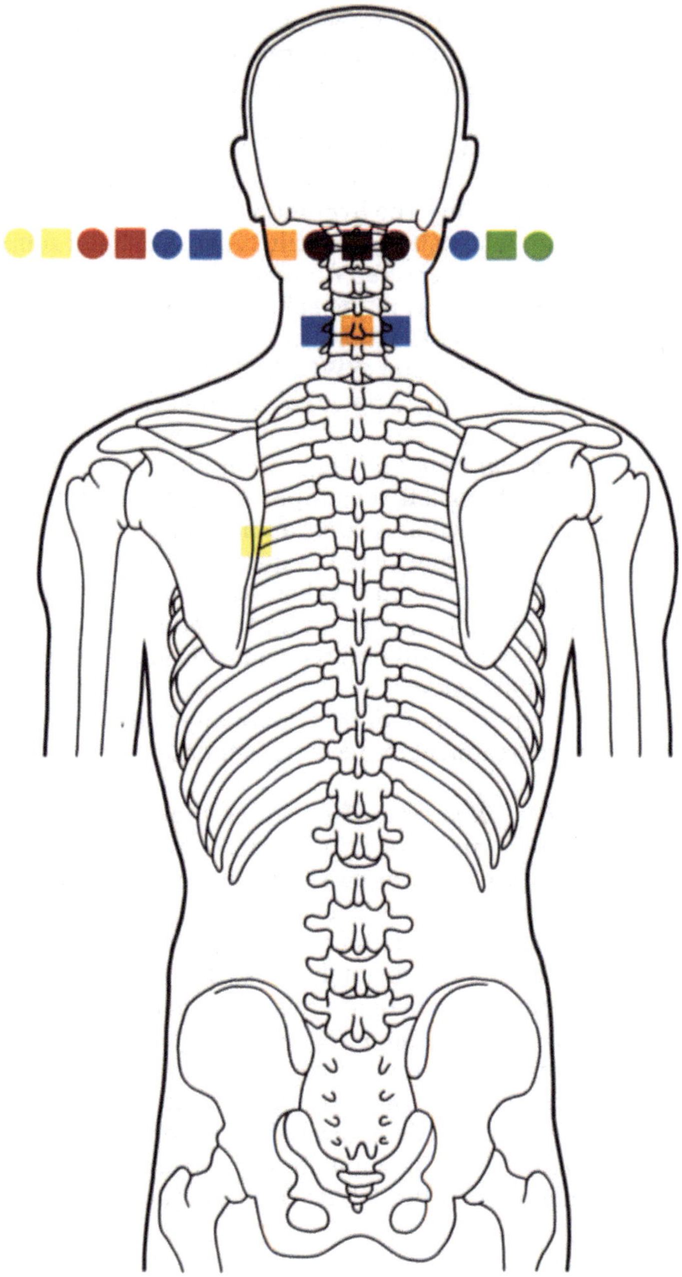

FRG: Cervico-thoracic junction/sacroiliac joint; muscle imbalance (shortening of postural muscles)

SWI: Bilateral hypomobility at C0-C1/C2-C3, left sacroiliac joint; increased tension in suboccipital muscles

UK: Hypomobility at C0-C1/C2-C3, increased muscle tension in suboccipital muscles

CZE/A: Hypomobility at C0-C1/C2-C3, increased muscle tension in suboccipital muscles

FRA: Hypomobility at C5-C6, increased tension in suboccipital muscles

Table 1. Patient 1, recommended treatment intervention

Examination protocol: International Seminar Week, 9-2-1983

Examiner: ______________________ Patient: No. 1

Recommended Treatment Plan

Area	Manipulation		Mobilization		MET	Muscle imbalance	Others
	L	R	L	R			
C0–C3	C C C C C	C C C C C	■	■	■ ■		■ Cervical Collar
C3–C6							
C7–T3	■						
T4–T8							
T8–L2							
L3–L5							
L5–SIJ	■ ■						

Use ☒ for recommended treatment; Ⓒ contraindication; ☐ main treatment modality

Remarks:

C = Every group considered manipulation as Contraindicated.

■	USA:	Cranial mobilization
■	FRG:	Muscle stretching
■	UK:	+ local anesthetic infiltration
■	CZE:	Muscle energy and traction

Patient 2: Sch. C., 40 Year Old Male

Chief Complaint:[2] Subsiding sciatica. The patient suffered from acute, recurrent, back pains within the past years. The last acute attack occurred two months before the date of this examination. The patient complains of pain radiating into the right buttock area and the right calf. The patient also reports occasional pain when coughing.

Social History:[3] The patient is a farmer and owner of a vineyard. Secured social and financial situation.

History of Chief Complaint: Sixteen years prior to this examination, the patient was injured in a car accident suffering a fractured pelvis (conservatively consolidated fracture of the pubic bone and the ischium). Five years ago sciatica pain appeared on the right side radiating into the margin of the right foot. Restricted mobility in the lumbar spine was noted. Also, mobility in the right hip was decreased and upon X-ray examination was diagnosed as a commencing arthrosis of the hip (coxarthrosis). These changes, however, were not viewed by the insurance company to be the result of the accident.
One year ago the deep tendon reflex was found absent as a result of an acute exacerbation of the sciatica. Therapy consisted then of local infiltration and peridural anesthesia with corticosteroids. Careful manipulation and mobilization exercises improved the symptoms of pain significantly.
Two months ago, the patient suffered an acute exacerbation during a horse-jumping exercise. The patient complains of pain in the right buttocks region, radiating to the right calf. The pain was worse with coughing and sneezing. Therapy consisted of shortwave treatment, in combination with careful mobilization at the lumbo-sacral regions and stretching of the dorsal back muscles and the hamstring muscles.

Laboratory Findings: Unremarkable.

X-ray Studies: The computer tomogram of the previous month indicates a small, medio-lateral disc herniation at L5–S1 on the right side (the computer tomogram of six months ago was normal).
X-ray studies of the lumbar spine, A.-P., and lateral views: the lumbosacral intervertebral disc is somewhat compressed. The distal surface of L_5 shows increased sclerotic changes. Otherwise, no abnormal degenerative changes are noted.

Problem: Is surgery indicated?

Examination Findings (Fig. 3): Every group reported a dysfunction at the right lumbo-sacral junction as the most significant finding. The dysfunction consists of decreased mobility, painful soft tissue changes (zone of irritations, increased tension in the soft tissues), shortening of the piriformis mus-

2 This information was available to the examining physicians for the first phase of the examination

3 The examiners were provided with this information only after completion of the original examination

cle and weakening of the gluteal muscles. The French and British groups indicate a secondary finding of hypomobility at the thoraco-lumbar junction whereas the American and German groups report a dysfunction in the left mid-thoracic region and the right cranio-cervical junction.

Therapeutic Plan (Table 2): None of the six groups indicated immediate surgical intervention for the small, mediolaterally herniated disc of L5–S1. Unanimously, the examiners would rather postpone such a procedure and observe the patient's further development and clinical symptoms.
The American, German, and Czechoslovakian-Austrian groups recommend as the primary treatment modality muscular rehabilitation along with soft tissue techniques (muscle energy techniques, mobilization) at the lumbo-sacral junction, as well as at the area of the second dysfunction, the midthoracic and upper-cervical spine. The Swiss group recommended only back exercises and back training. The French school recommends the wearing of a lumbar-pelvic plaster-of-Paris jacket for three weeks, upon which careful manipulation can be employed. If these procedures did not lead to improvement, surgical procedures would be indicated.
The British group suggested primarily specific manipulation to the thoraco-lumbar junction followed by epidural anesthesia. If the results prove to be unsatisfactory, however, surgical intervention would have to be considered.

Authors' Remarks: This 40-year-old patient seems to be a typical representative of a group of patients with chronic disc pathologies who frequently present the physician with difficulties not only in regard to making a precise diagnosis but also in regard to the therapeutic interventions.
Patients who demonstrate clear radicular symptoms with acute severe sciatica and whose herniated disc can be demonstrated radiologically seem to show better operative results than patients with chronically recurring, non-distinct pain syndromes or alternating radicular symptoms (Dvorak and Gauchat, unpublished observations).
These empirical findings seem to correlate well with the rather cautious approach of the physicians in this study, since they did not choose surgical procedures as their first choice of treatment intervention. Rather, exercises for the back or home training in conjunction with the supportive mobilization of the the lumbo-sacral junction were the major treatment form. It is interesting to note that four groups considered the dysfunctions at the thoraco-lumbar junction, the mid-thoracic region and the upper-cervical spine to be secondary to the dysfunction in the lumbo-sacral region. These findings may be the result of the spondylogenic reflex syndrome.

Fig. 3. Patient 2: Sch. C., 40 year old male; major findings

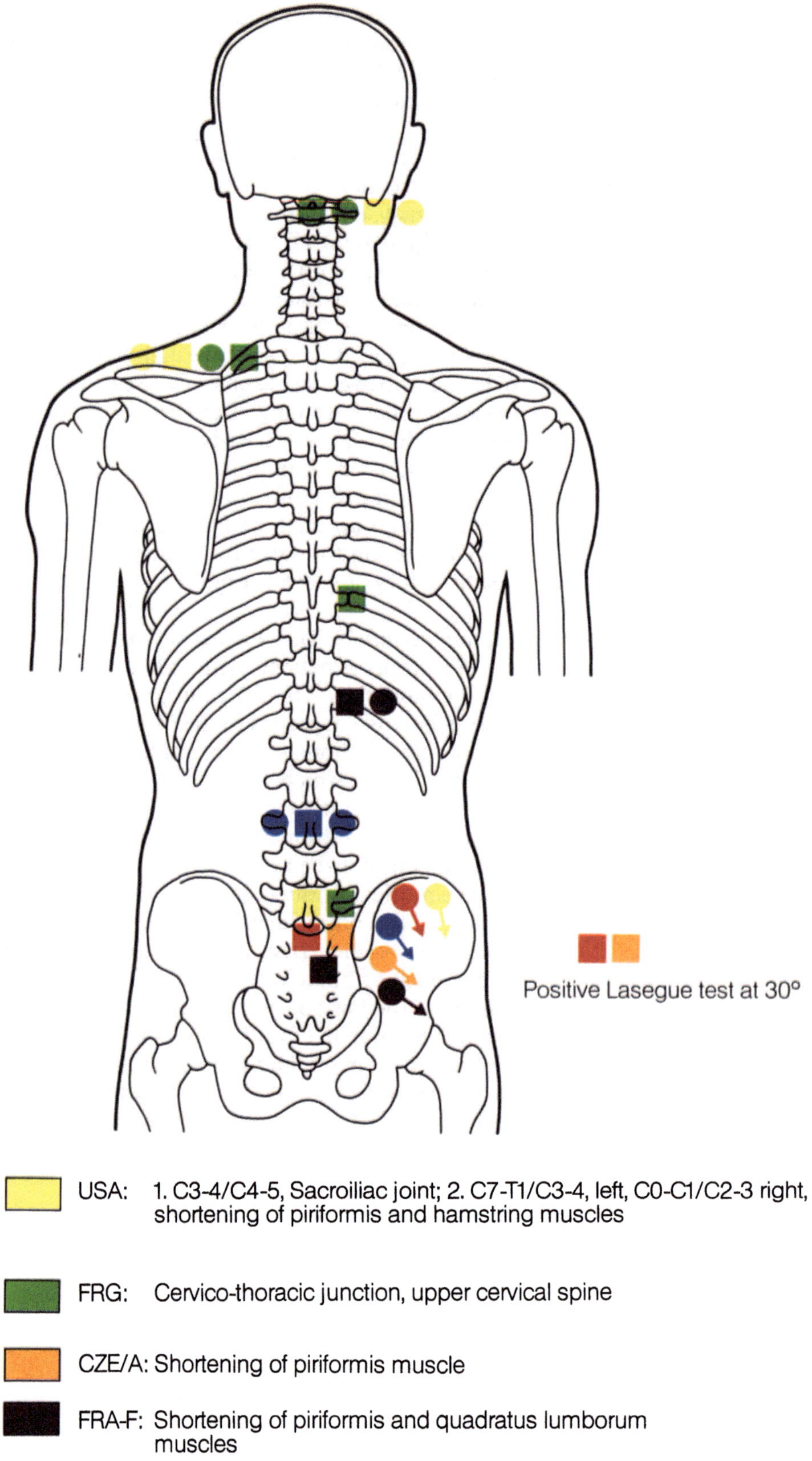

Table 2. Patient 2, recommended treatment intervention

Examination protocol: International Seminar Week, 9-2-1983

Examiner: ______________________ Patient: No. 2

Recommended Treatment Plan

Area	Manipulation		Mobilization		MET	Muscle imbalance	Others
	L	R	L	R			
C0–C3	■ [green]	■ [green]			■ [yellow]		
C3–C6							
C7–T3	■ [green]				■ [yellow]		
T4–T8							
T8–L2	■ [green] ■ [blue]	■ [green] ■ [blue]					
L3–L5			■ [dark brown]	■ [dark brown]			■ [green] Physical therapy ■ [red] Posture training. ■ [dark brown] Corset
L5–SIJ					■ [yellow]		

Use ☒ for recommended treatment; 🄲 contraindication; ☐ main treatment modality

Remarks:

- [yellow] USA: Muscle rehabilitation, treatment directed towards secondary changes, no immediate surgical intervention
- [green] FRG: Physical therapy, stretching of lumbosacral muscles; treatment of secondary changes; manipulation (thoracic but not cervical spine)
- [red] SWI-CH: Back training; surgical intervention not indicated since there is no paresis present
- [blue] UK: Manipulation, no indication for operation because of missing pareses
- [orange] CZE/A: If manipulation does not lead to improvement, surgical intervention is indicated
- [dark brown] FRA-F: Plaster corset for 3 weeks followed by manipulation; if no improvement surgical procedures are indicated

Patient 3: D. A., 53 Year Old Female

Chief Complaint:[4] Following a car accident seven years ago, the patient has been complaining of repeated pain attacks and decreased ability to flex her spine. The pain radiates into the shoulder blade regions and occasionally into the lumbar spine, and quite frequently the pain between the shoulder blades wakes the patient up at night. Minimal manual labor, such as cleaning windows provoke pain.

Social History: The patient, a former teacher, is presently a housewife.

History of Chief Complaint: The first accident, which took place in 1976, was a head-on collision. The patient was wearing a seat belt. With a latency period of approximately six hours, a torticollis developed with restricted motion in the cervical spine. In the years following, the patient underwent several forms of treatment, among them manual therapy, acupuncture, massages, and drug therapy. Four years after the accident the patient was almost symptom free and was fit for work.
A second accident occurred three years ago (the patient had thus been symptom free for one year). At high speed, the patient who wore her seat belt collided with a truck next to her on the highway. The car was thrown back and forth several times between the left and right guard rail. The patient reports amnesia of the collision, and she suffered minor lacerations and contusions. The car was irreparably damaged.
Immediately upon gaining consciousness, the patient noticed great thoracic pain especially when breathing and persistent pain in the neck region. X-ray studies suggested a possible fracture of the ninth thoracic vertebra, but could not be confirmed unequivocally.
The patient received a neck collar but due to allergic reactions she was not able to wear the collar permanently.
Because of the neck pains, the patient was basically confined to a lying position for a considerable amount of time. Mobilizing exercises were extremely painful.
At the time of this examination the patient complained of pressure sensation above the eyes and at the occiput which was exacerbated when holding the head in flexion for a longer period of time. Flexion further caused pain in the lower cervical spine and the mid-thoracic spine.

Laboratory Findings: Normal.

X-ray Studies: The cervical spine was X-rayed in the A. P. and lateral positions, including maximal flexion and extension. The intervertebral discs C4–5 and C5–6 are somewhat compressed, and a few spondylophytes were found within the bodies of C3, C4, and C5 anteriorly and possibly posteriorly. Limited arthrosis in the apophyseal joints of C5 and C6 was observed. No indication of instability.
The lateral view of the thoracic spine revealed the following: small wedge-shaped deformation of the ninth thoracic body with the anterior portion of

4 This information was available to the examining physicians during the first phase of the examination

the vertebral body being compressed 3 mm. The bony structure of the body appears to be normal, and no reactive degenerative ossifications in the soft tissues are noted. The remaining thoracic spine is unremarkable.

Problem:
- Determination of a rehabilitation plan.
- Is manual therapy to the mid-cervical spine indicated?
- Which, if any, diagnostic procedures should be employed further?

Examination Findings (Fig. 4): The examiners of all six groups reported as one of the three major findings the one elicited in the mid-thoracic region. The segmental and regional dysfunctions of the mid-thoracic spine were diagnosed by utilizing motion testing or soft tissue evaluation (zone of irritation, myotendinosis). Furthermore, the Czechoslovakian, British, French, and Swiss groups were in agreement in regard to findings in the cervico-thoracic junction; the representatives from Czechoslavakia, United Kingdom, USA, and Germany noticed a functional hypomobility in the cranio-cervical junction. All six groups reported bilateral muscle tension in the sub-occipital musculature.
The Swiss, American, German, and English representatives further indicated a dysfunction in the lumbo-sacral junction which they considered to be secondary to the primary dysfunction in the cervical and thoracic spine. The Czechoslovakian-Austrian group called attention to the pathological respiration movements of the patient, i.e., elevated ribs during expiration.

Therapeutic Plan (Table 3): Each of the six groups sees an indication for specific treatment at the cervical spine, where soft tissue techniques such as muscle energy techniques or soft mobilization techniques are the preferred modality. The Swiss participants viewed manipulation and mobilization as contraindicated in the patient and would only treat the tense muscles in the sub-occipital and cervical regions with muscle stretch techniques.
Only the French group would consider manipulation at the mid-cervical and lower cervical spine; upon the completion of manipulative therapy they suggest the wearing of a stabilizing neck collar for three weeks.
There was considerable agreement in regard to the therapeutic intervention at the mid-thoracic spine and the lumbo-sacral junction. Specific manipulation or mobilization techniques were suggested for these two regions, accompanied by appropriate treatment procedures to improve muscular imbalance.
The Czechoslovakian group further recommends breathing exercises. In the event manipulative or mobilizing therapy does not lead to the desired result, the British members would resort to local infiltration of the apophyseal joints at the cervical and thoracic spine with adjunctive transcutaneous stimulation.

Authors' Remarks: Due to its chronic nature – the result of two whiplash injuries affecting the cervical spine as well as the possible result of a contusion at the mid-thoracic spine – this case offers a wide spectrum of clinical findings. In that regard, it is remarkable that the group as a whole reported findings localized to the region of the mid-thoracic spine. Other regions of interest, such as the cervico-thoracic junction, the upper cervical spine and in particular the lumbo-sacral junction, which presented the patient with relatively few symptoms, however, were subject to major agreement. The exam-

Fig. 4. Patient 3: D. A., 53 year old female; major findings

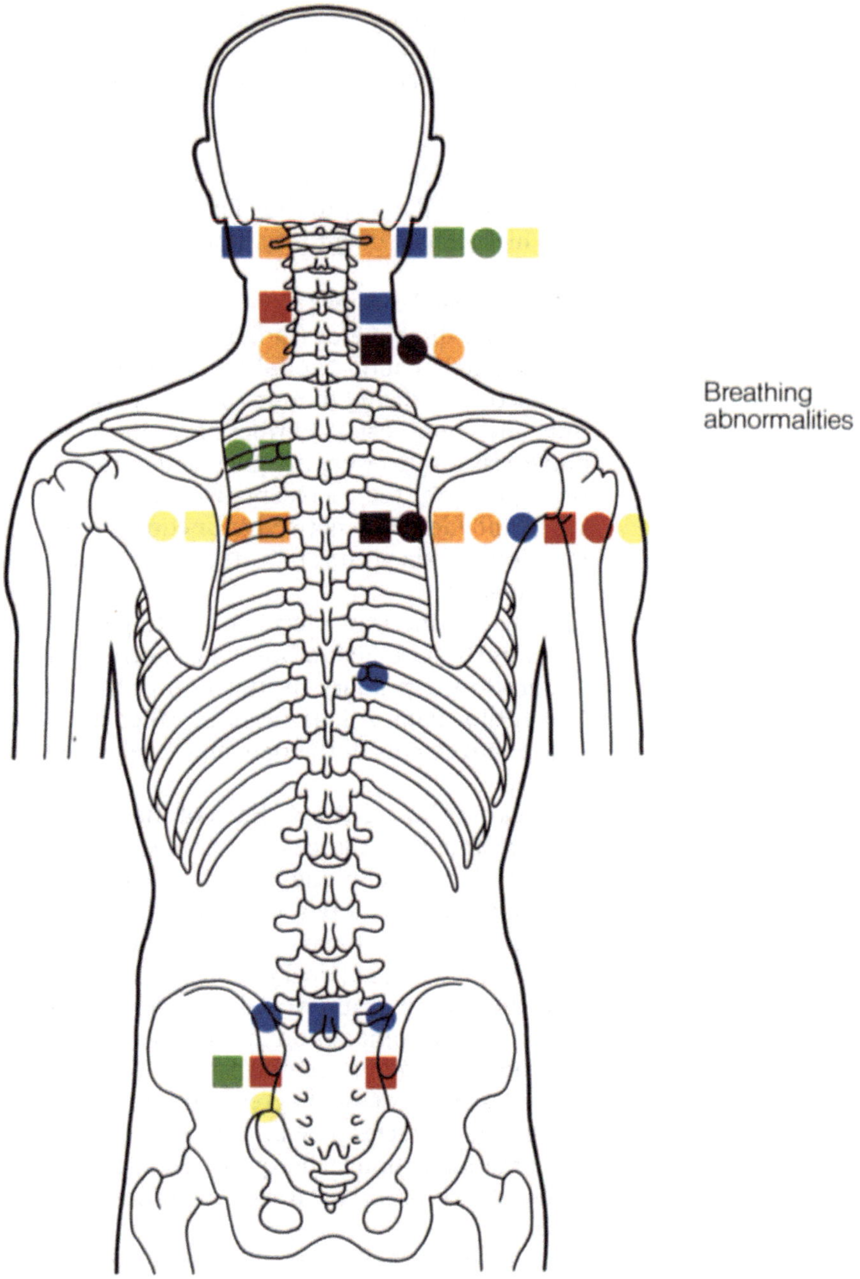

Yellow	USA:	Suboccipital muscles show increased tension
Green	FRG:	Muscle imbalance
Red	SWI-CH:	Suboccipital muscles show increased tension
Blue	UK:	Hypomobility-entire cervical spine
Orange	CZE/A:	Breathing abnormalities, muscle imbalance
Black	FRA-F:	Thoracic spine; secondary changes

Table 3. Patient 3, recommended treatment intervention

Examination protocol: International Seminar Week, 9-2-1983

Examiner: __________ Patient: No. 3

Recommended Treatment Plan

Area	Manipulation		Mobilization		MET	Muscle imbalance	Others
	L	R	L	R			
CO–C3				green, orange	yellow, green, orange		
C3–C6	blue (C)	black (C)	blue	orange (C)	orange	red-brown	
C7–T3					green		
T4–T8	yellow, black	yellow, black	orange	orange	yellow, orange		
T8–L2							
L3–L5							
L5–SIJ	red-brown, blue	red-brown, blue			yellow	green	

Use ☒ for recommended treatment; Ⓒ contraindication; ☐ main treatment modality

Remarks:

[yellow] USA: Concentrate on mid thoracic spine, muscle stretching, some cervical spine treatment

[green] FRG: Treatment to improve muscle imbalance

[blue] UK: Soft mobilization directed towards cervical spine and local infiltration of its apophyseal joints, thoracic spine physical therapy

[orange] CZE: Muscle stretching, improvement of respiration

[black] FRA-F: Following cervical spine manipulation, the wearing of the of a collare for 3 weeks at night is recommended

iners considered these findings to be secondary and related to the spondylogenic syndrome.

The different therapeutic approach is a reflection of the varying viewpoints in the different schools. The representatives from France and Switzerland held exactly opposing points of view. While the French school would use manipulation at the mid-cervical spine, the Swiss school views such a treatment as contraindicated and would no go beyond muscle-stretch techniques for treatment of the tightened muscles.

All other groups recommended careful mobilization or muscle energy techniques. Overall, it seems that soft tissue techniques are preferred over the classical manipulation with impulse (thrust) when treating a patient with chronic, post-traumatic involvement of the cervical spine.

Since the X-ray studies did not unequivocally indicate a fracture in the mid-thoracic spine, some examiners (USA, F, CZE) would perform manipulation or mobilization at this region.

Furthermore, the representatives from Switzerland, the UK, the USA, and Germany would treat the secondary dysfunction at the sacroiliac joint with manipulation or mobilization techniques.

Patient 4, G. C., 35 Year Old Male

Chief Complaint[5]: The patient complains of recurrent back pain which is exacerbated with loading. The pain at times radiates into the right leg and occasionally into the cervical spine region.

Social History[6]: The patient is a mechanical engineer working primarily in the office. Good family situation.

History of Chief Complaint: When serving in the military six years prior to this visit, the first pain attacks appeared following a slight trauma when he was lifting heavy objects. From the beginning the pain has radiated into the patient's right leg. Neurological examination three years ago found an absent achilles-tendon reflex. One year later, the reflexes of the lower extremities were symmetrical.
Conservative treatment during acute painful periods showed good results within the past six years. Most often a few manipulations sufficed to relieve the patient's symptoms. One year ago, intensive physical therapy such as heat treatments and muscle stretching became necessary, however. The patient was always fit for work, and there were no insurance problems.

Laboratory: Unremarkable.

X-rays: A.-P. and lateral views of the lumbar spine showed normal intervetebral spaces, and intact bony structures.

Problem: This case presents few problems. Manipulation was always able to alleviate the acute painful attacks. A minute disk-herniation at L5-S1 is possibly present. For the patient, the major problem is the reduced ability to perform physical activities.

Examination Findings (Fig. 5): Every group, with the exception of the French, reports a main finding in the sacroiliac region. The findings were described as hypomobility with concomitant myotendinosis in the gluteal musculature (gluteus maximus muscle, piriformis muscle). In addition to hypomobility, the Swiss and British groups report tender points (zones of irritation, trigger points) at the level of the sacroiliac joints. The French group, indicates as their most significant finding a dysfunction at the segments of L3–L4, L5–S1, and T12.
Every group, again with the exception of the French, report secondary findings consisting of localized changes at the right upper cervical spine, which are described as hypomobility with myotendinoses of the suboccipital muscles.
The representatives from Switzerland, the UK, Germany, and France elicited a regional dysfunction in the cervico-thoracic junction.
The American and German representatives furthermore noticed a right sided segmental dysfunction at level T12 and L2.
Every group described a muscular imbalance in the gluteal region with shortening in the postural and weakness in the phasic muscles.

5 This information was available to the examiners during the first phase of the study
6 This information was given to the examiners upon completion of the examination protocol

Therapeutic Plan (Table 5): As suggested by the physicians from Switzerland, the USA, Czechoslovakia and West Germany the first line of treatment should consist of specific, well localized manipulation, mobilization and muscle energy techniques directed towards the lumbo-sacral junction. The French group recommended specific manipulation at the lower lumbar region. There was agreement among all the groups in regard to the secondary dysfunction at the cervico-thoracic junction and the upper cervical spine, for which manipulation and mobilization techniques were recommended.
In the event that this form of treatment proves to be unsuccessful, the British group would employ epidural anesthesia.

Authors' Remarks: All physicians, with the exception of the representatives from France, considered the presence of the hypomobility in the right sacroiliac joint as the major problem. Thus, the majority of the investigators would utilize manipulation techniques directed towards the right sacroiliac joint as their primary therapeutic modality. The lumboradicular symptoms from one year ago, the absent achilles-tendon-reflex and pain radiating into the dermatome S1 were not considered to be contraindicated to manipulation at the sacroiliac joints.

Fig. 5. Patient 4: G. C., 35 year old male; major findings

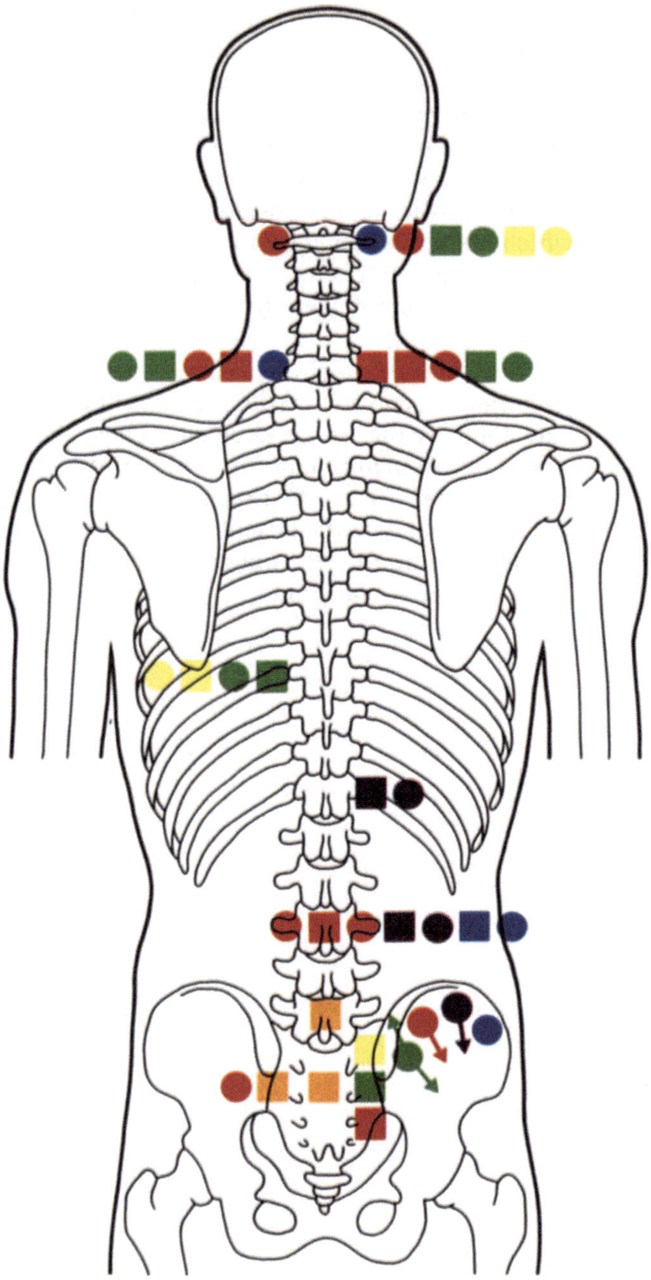

- USA: Tension in suboccipital muscles, iliopsoas and piriformis muscle
- FRG: Iliopsoas and suboccipital muscles; shortened hamstring muscles
- SWI-CH: Piriformis muscle; weakened gluteal muscles
- UK: Pain referred to gluteal region
- FRA-F: Piriformis muscle

Table 4. Patient 4, recommended treatment intervention

Examination protocol: International Seminar Week, 9-2-1983

Examiner: ______________ Patient: No. 4

Recommended Treatment Plan

Area	Manipulation		Mobilization		MET	Muscle imbalance	Others
	L	R	L	R			
C0–C3	[blue]			[green]	[yellow]		
C3–C6		[black]					
C7–T3	[red]	[green] [red]					
T4–T8							
T8–L2	[green] [blue]	[yellow]					
L3–L5	[orange]	[orange] [black]					
L5–SIJ		[yellow] [green]		[red]	[yellow]	[green]	

Use ☒ for recommended treatment; Ⓒ contraindication; ☐ main treatment modality

Remarks:

[blue] UK: Epidural anesthesia

Patient No. 5: M. U., 42 Year Old Female

Chief Complaint[7]: The patient complains of pain in the shoulder and neck regions. The pain is exacerbated when there is loading or strain in these areas. At the present time, the most painful area is the inter-scapular region. The patient has responded well to antirheumatic drug therapy.

Social History[8]: The patient is married and has two children. Before an accident eight years ago, the patient had been working full time as an executive secretary. Five years prior to this examination (after the car accident) she had personal problems at home as well as at her job, underwent a divorce, and unresolved insurance and medical problems existed. Presently the patient feels the situation has significantly improved.

History of Chief Complaint: The patient was involved in a car collision eight years prior to this examination. She was not unconscious. In the hospital, she was immobilized for a short period of time. In the weeks and months following the car accident, neck pains and headaches developed, as did non-specific vertigo and concomitant temporary vomiting. The pain radiated into both shoulder blade regions. One year after the accident, six specific manipulations at the C2–C3 region were effected by an experienced rheumatologist trained in manual therapy. After the first two manipulative procedures the patient had virtually no complaints. Additional four manipulative interventions, however, showed no further improvement, and, the original symptoms (vertigo, vomiting, headaches, and severe neck pain) actually reappeared. Upon functional X-ray examination of the cervical spine, instability at the atlanto-axial joints became evident and was consequently stabilized with spondylodesis prior to which the cervical spine had been successfully immobilized by a Minerva jacket for six weeks. This procedure seemed to have almost completely resolved the vertigo attacks, vomiting, and the pain experienced in the neck region. Within the past two to three years the patient has been complaining about increasing neck pains radiating into the thoracic spine region. Without informing her physician she was treated by another rheumatologist who also had training in manual therapy and who must have applied great force, since the patient perceived a "cracking noise." The patient vomited for several hours after the treatment. As a result of the painful exacerbation in the patient's neck and thoracic spine the upper cercival joints, the thoracic spine and the lumbosacral junction were specifically mobilized this time by the attending rheumatologist. Both the neck and back pains disappeared, the pain in the mid-thoracic spine, however, persisted.

Laboratory Findings: Unremarkable.

X-ray Studies: A.-P. and lateral views of the cervical spine, including those at maximal flexion and extension positions showed a stable posterior spondylodesis at C1–2 with metal wire in position.
The intervertebral disk of C3–4 and C4–5 are somewhat compressed but noticable spondylosis formation can be seen. The functional view shows that the spondylodesis at C1–2 is completely stable and the remaining segments including C0–C1 can move normally.

---

7 This information was available to the examiners during the first phase of the study
8 This information was given to the examiners upon completion of the examination protocol

Problem: It is necessary to start a medium-term rehabilitation program. Apparently secondary spondylogenic phenomena have appeared, the interpretation of which seems difficult. Problems regarding insurance compensation do not exist.

Examination Findings (Fig. 6): All operators diagnosed a hypomobile area in the upper cervical spine, the cervico-thoracic junction and the mid-thoracic spine, along with myotendinoses of the suboccipital musculature. In the functional examination of the musculature, shortening of the trapezius muscle, levator scapulae and rhomboid muscles were described by all groups. Secondary findings such as a regional dysfunction in the thoraco-lumbar junction were noted by the American and German groups, whereas the British, Swiss and German groups reported a disturbance in the sacroiliac joint as well.

Therapeutic Plan (Table 5): As noted by all six groups, manipulation or mobilization to the upper cervical spine region is clearly contraindicated. Different viewpoints were expressed regarding the treatment of the lower regions of the vertebral column. The French group recommended manipulation to the lower cervical spine, whereas the Czechoslovakian representative would only treat this region by muscle energy technique. The Swiss participants suggested mobilization of the cervico-thoracic junction. Even though differing in the treatment modality, all groups, with the exception of the British, thought that the mid-thoracic spine needed treatment; Switzerland would use manipulation, France and West Germany prefer mobilization, and the USA and Czechoslovakia would empoly muscle energy techniques.
The representatives from Germany and Czechoslovakia recommended mobilization at the thoraco-lumbar junction, the British manipulation at the lower lumbar spine, whereas the German and Swiss operators proposed manipulation to the sacroiliac joints.
For treatment of painful acute exacerbations the British group recommends local lidocaine infiltration into the patient's cervico-thoracic junction.

Authors' Remarks: The authors used this case as a "diagnostic trap." The scar of the posterior spondylodesis is in close proximity of the patient's hairline. The examining physician not familiar with the history would most probably miss this scar unless he pays particular attention to this region. It is thus remarkable that without exception every group detected the hypomobile area and muscular myotendinosis in this particular region.
There was general agreement regarding the findings at the cervico-thoracic junction and the mid-thoracic spine. In these regions as well, the diagnosis that was brought forth consisted of hypomobility and shortening of the shoulder and neck muscles.
Four groups described secondary dysfunctions, namely those of hypomobility in the thoraco-lumbar junction and dysfunctions in the sacroiliac joints. Though not surprising, it is encouraging to note that with knowledge of the detailed history every group would consider such procedures as manipulation or mobilization to the upper cervical spine as contraindicated.

Fig. 6. Patient 5: M. U., 42 year old female; major findings

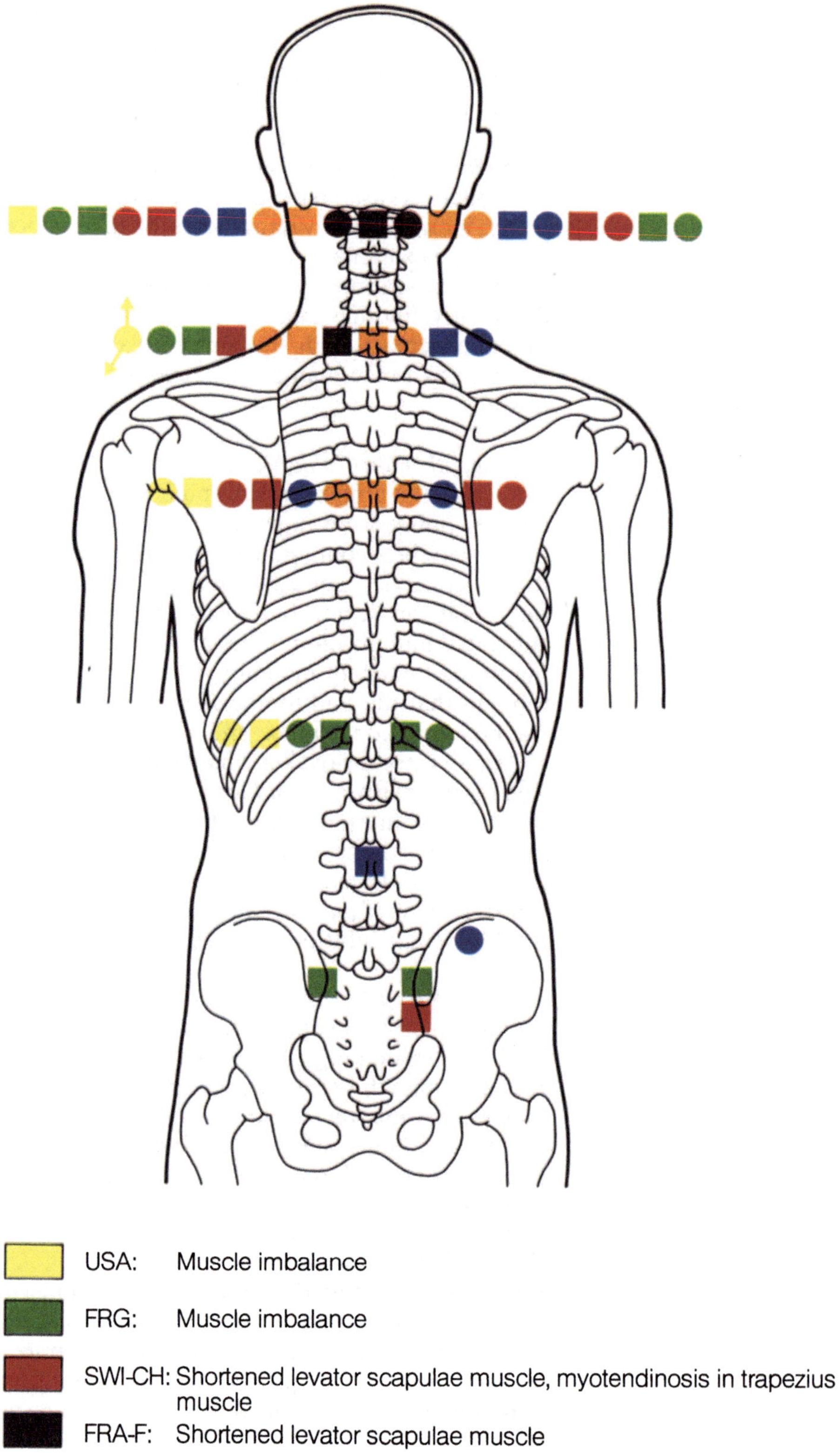

Table 5. Patient 5, recommended treatment intervention (including contra indication)

Examination protocol: International Seminar Week, 9-2-1983

Examiner: ______________________ Patient: No. 5

Recommended Treatment Plan

Area	Manipulation		Mobilization		MET	Muscle imbalance	Others
	L	R	L	R			
C0–C3	C C C C C C	C C C C C C	C	C			■ cranial
C3–C6	■		■	■	■		■ injection
C7–T3			■	■			
T4–T8		■	■ ■	■ ■	■ ■		
T8–L2			■	■	■		
L3–L5	■	■					
L5–SIJ	■ ■	■ ■	■	■			

Use ☒ for recommended treatment; [C] contraindication; ☐ main treatment modality

Remarks:

■ UK: Local infiltration with lidocaine in the apophyseal joints of C4–T2

Patient 6: H. R., 23 Year Old Male

Chief Complaint:[9] The patient suffers primarily from back pain that does not respond to therapy. The pain is exacerbated when loading is abnormal or assuming wrong body posture. The pain does not radiate appreciably into the legs.

Social History[10]: The patient works as a clerk, with no physical labor involved. The patient only exercises minimally.

History of Chief Complaint: The present back pains had started during military service three years ago, as a result of which the patient was reassigned to office duties. Radicular failure could not be determined. The left sacroiliac joint indicated a somatic dysfunction at times. Zones of irritation appear in the region of the thoraco-lumbar junction when greater lumbar lordosis is introduced. The attending rheumatologist conducted several specific manipulations, passive mobilization procedures for the sacroiliac joints and muscle stretching of the hamstring and posterior back muscles.

Laboratory Findings: Unremarkable.

X-ray Studies: The A.-P. and lateral views of the lumbar spine revealed the following: The intervertebral disk spaces show no abnormalities, and the sacroiliac joints have normal contours. Degenerative changes are not noted. The bony structures are intact.

Problem: There is discrepancy between the patient's symptoms and the objective findings. As reported by the patient the pain seems not to respond to therapy. Are we confronted with psychosomatic back pain?

Examination Findings (Fig. 7: All six groups diagnosed a hypomobile area of soft tissue changes in the region of the lumbo-sacral junction. The American, Czechoslovakian, and Swiss groups stressed the presence of a bilateral dysfunction at the sacroiliac joint. A secondary finding, that of hypomobility in the region of the upper cervical joints, is described by the Czechoslovakian, American, German, and Swiss groups.
The English group reported no restriction whatsoever regarding the mobility of the total spine, but found soft tissue changes in the lumbo-sacral region. The German group diagnosed a significant muscular imbalance in the region of the thoraco-lumbar junction.

Therapeutic Plan (Table 6): The Czechoslovakian, American, German, and Swiss groups would treat the sacroiliac joints with specific, localized mobilization or muscle energy techniques, whereas the French group recommends specific manipulation to the upper lumbar spine. The American and German groups would then treat the cervico-thoracic junction and the upper cervical spine employing mobilization. The English group suggests local infiltration of the lumbar apophyseal joints.

9 The examiners were provided with this information for the first step of the examination
10 The following information was provided upon completion of the examination protocol

None of the groups reported the possibility of aggravation of the patient's neurotic attitude based on the symptoms provided.

Authors' Remarks: The authors were unable to determine the extent to which the patient's symptoms could be ascribed to a segmental dysfunction, or whether this patient should be considered a representative of a group of patients who have constant pain but no major psychopathology.

As is generally known, it is extremely difficult to differentiate this type of patient from

- conversion-neurotic-hysteric patients, who rather unconsciously want to gain advantage by imitating a disease
- those patients who exceedingly exaggerate their symptoms, hoping to obtain a pension or receive greater attention of the environment, etc. (secondary gain patient).
- true malingerers.

Even though all the examiners located pathological findings at the area of the lumbo-sacral junction, one cannot clearly distinguish the extent to which the patient deceived the operators during their examination procedures by volunteering information about pain or exhibiting a guarded reaction. Conversely, it cannot be decided whether a functional disturbances at the sacro-iliac joint was the real cause of the pain reported by the patient. Thus, one is unable to come to a final, clearcut conclusion in this case.

Fig. 7. Patient 6: H. R., 23 year old male; major findings

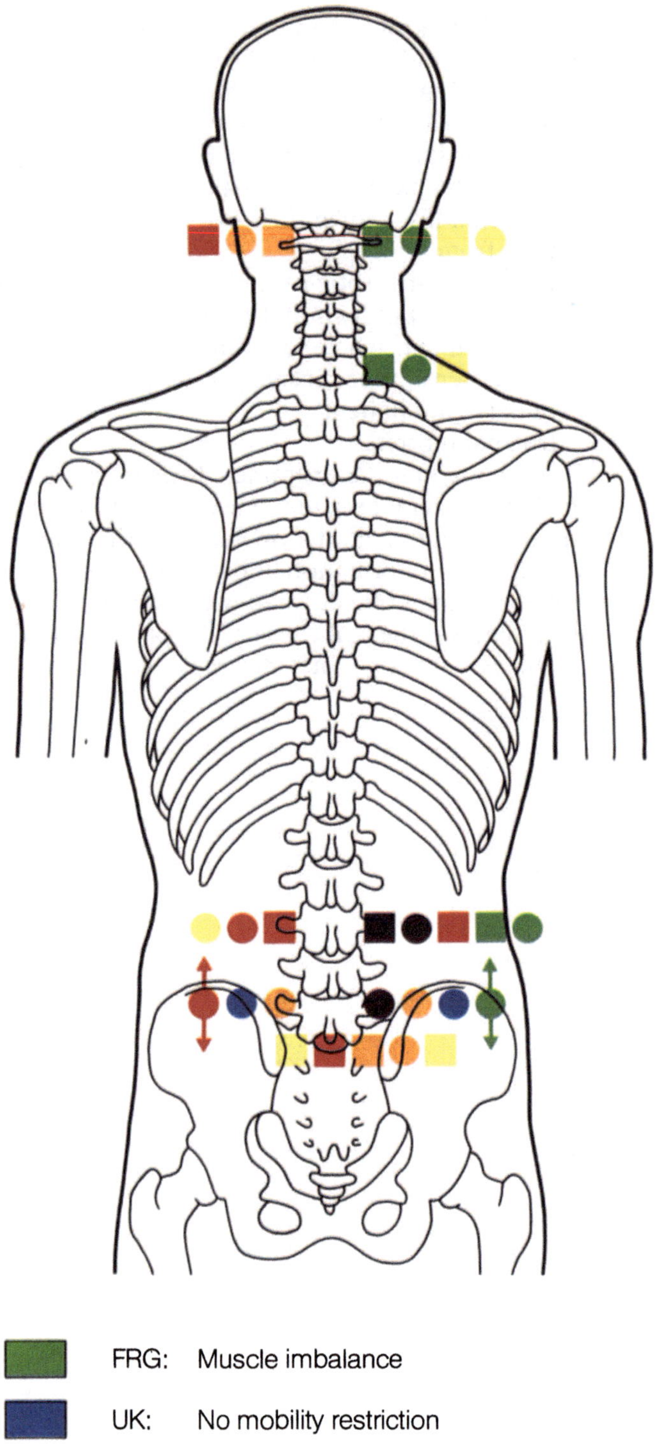

Table 6. Patient 6, recommended treatment intervention

Examination protocol: International Seminar Week, 9-2-1983

Examiner: ____________ Patient: No. 6

Recommended Treatment Plan

Area	Manipulation		Mobilization		MET	Muscle imbalance	Others
	L	R	L	R			
C0–C3			■ ■	■ ■			
C3–C6			■	■			
C7–T3					■		
T4–T8							
T8–L2		■				■	
L3–L5				■	■	■ ■	■ injection
L5–SIJ				■	■ ■		

Use ☒ for recommended treatment; Ⓒ contraindication; ☐ main treatment modality

Remarks:

■ SWI-CH: Exercises to improve stability; no immediate manipulation

■ UK: Local infiltration

Chapter 3

Cranio-Cervical Junction

Participants:

Australia (AUS): C. Winer
France (F): P. Juvin
Switzerland (SWI):
H. Baumgartner,
F. Schönenberger
United Kingdom (UK):
L. Burn
USA: R. Kappler
West Germany (FRG):
K. Seifert, H. D. Wolff

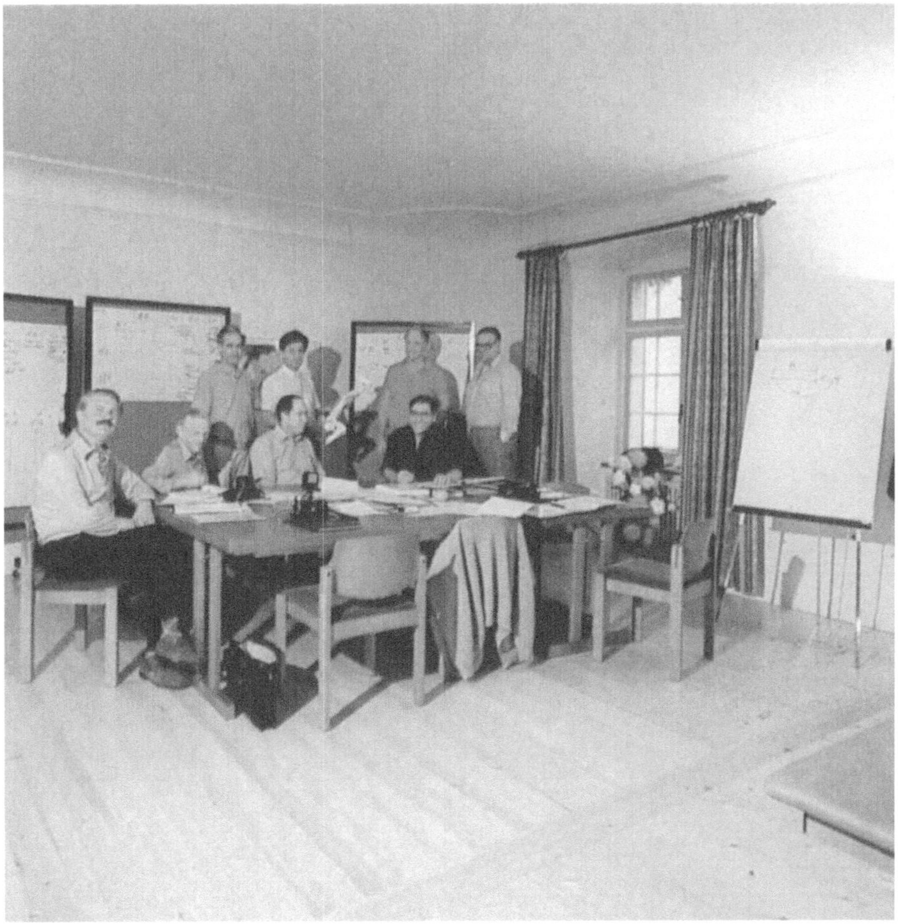

3.1 General Remarks Concerning the Cranio-Cervical Junction

3.1.1 General Considerations

3.1.1.1 To What Extent Is the Diagnosis Influenced by the Appearance of Pain or Decreased Mobility?

The British and French representatives share the viewpoint that the appearance of pain is more significant in the diagnositic process, whereas the Swiss and German representatives consider pain and decreased mobility to be of equal importance. For the American and Australian representatives, restricted joint mobility is of greatest importance.

3.1.1.2 How Significant Is the Sequence of Treatment in the Pain-free Direction?

While the French and British participants consider both the diagnostic and therapeutic manipulation in the pain-free direction as their major significant criterion, the representatives from the other countries do not share this strict approach. This, however, is valid only for the gross examination but not for the segmental examination and treatment.

3.1.1.3 What Is the Cause of Pain?

The French participants are convinced that one always deals with radicular pain (pain syndrome of the dorsal rami of the nerve roots). The other participants make a distinction between primary radicular pain and the pain manifestation due to the stimulation of the nociceptors in the fibrous joint capsules. One can interpret referred pain in a similar manner, which is probably the result of reflexogenic action.
The French school furthermore believes that a mechanical disturbance in a spinal segment with the consequent radicular symptoms is the primary cause, whereas the other countries view it as a complex pathogenic disturbance.

3.1.1.4 Is the Patient To Be Treated in the Sitting or Standing Position?

The majority of the group recommens treatment of the suboccipital region with the patient supine. The Swiss representatives, however, believe that examination of the patient in the sitting position does not restrict their diagnostic assessment nor the examination procedures themselves. Germany utilizes both the sitting and lying positions consistently because of the importance that is attached to the tension relationships of the small suboccupital muscles, whose tone increases significantly when the patient is sitting.

3.1.1.5 Mobilization or Manipulation?

For the USA, this issue depends on certain circumstances. That is, if the case is more severe, mobilization would be used primarily. With the case being less severe, manipulation would be the first approach. The representatives from England and France use manipulation unless certain contraindications exist (primarily in regard to the vertebral artery).
For the suboccipital region, the Swiss prefer mobilizing techniques to manipulative procedures which use impulse (thrust) so as to prevent further complications at the upper cervical spine.
The German group considers manipulative and mobilizing techniques to be of equal importance.
In Australia mobilization is given primacy, first for patient comfort and secondly for risk reduction.

3.1.1.6 X-ray Studies and Their Application

It was agreed that the conventional x-ray studies of the cervical spine (A.-P. and lateral views) do not contribute much to the functional diagnosis and therapeutic approach. The primary use of radiological studies is to determine contraindications such osteoporosis, tumors, de- and malformations, as well as highly degenerative changes. It is naturally understood that post-traumatic pain in the neck region requires an indepth radiological evaluation.
Functional examinations such as lateral and A.-P. views (flexion-extension, sidebending) can sometimes provide valuable information as to which therapeutic procedure is to be applied.

3.1.1.7 Can a Dysfunction in the Cranio-Cervical Junction Influence Other Parts of the Musculo-Skeletal System or the Extremities?

The French participants feel that functional disturbances influence only adjoining spinal segments and are thus considered localized with no further spread. The rest of the group did not agree with this opinion and believes that the clinical distribution resulting from such disturbances is generally more widespread, with the possibility of influencing the extremities. Dysfunctions affecting distant regions are assumed to be related to referred pain or to be reflexogenic reactions with irritation of the fibrous joint capsule.

3.1.2 Diagnosis

The representatives from the different countries attribute different significance to the individual diagnostic procedures such as the "pincer rouler" (skin rolling), the modality of suboccipital muscle palpation and their respective attachments. The German and Swiss representatives place great emphasis on both the functional and palpatory examination of the suboccipital musculature. The Swiss further call attention to the distant, systematized myotendinoses, which are considered to be the result of the spondylogenic reflex syndrome.

The most important diagnostic criteria for the Swiss are those soft tissue changes that are related neither to tendons nor muscles and that are considered to be the surface manifestation of a segmental dysfunction (segmental zone of irritation). Everyone felt that regional motion evaluation is an essential test as are the passive screening tests that assess segmental mobility. France alone considers these particular tests to be of little value.
The representatives from Germany, Switzerland, and Australia do evaluate the atlanto-occipital mobility including the axial end rotation (joint play) between atlas and the occiput.
The Swiss school further concentrates on the rotatory movement between the atlas and axis when the cervical spine is maximally flexed. The normal value for some such motion is 45° to either side. Axial rotation in the segment C2–C3 is tested best when the head is inclined (flexed forward) while the cervical spine is extended. One measures the range of motion by palpating the movement of the spinous processes during this motion.
Functional length testing of the shoulder and neck muscles (descending trapezius muscle, levator scapulae muscle, semispinalis capitis muscle) is routinely done in all countries except in France and the United Kingdom.

3.1.3 Treatment

With regard to soft tissue treatment and that of the muscular imbalance, there was agreement among the American, German, and Swiss representatives, who place great emphasis on the stretching of the shortened and strengthening of the weakened muscles. There was unity in regard to the value of manipulation and mobilization without impulse (no thrust). The Swiss, however, stressed that they treat the patient sitting, in contrast to all the other schools who prefer the patient lying.

3.2 Biomechanics of the Cranio-Cervical Junction

The first problem the group had to cope with was whether it should restrict itself to the cranial-vertebral junction and inferior cervical joints or include the cranium as was suggested by the American osteopathic physician.
It was decided to concentrate on problems dealing with the upper cervical spine and the atlanto-occipital junction only.

3.2.1 Atlanto-Occipital Joint

The articulation between the skull and the atlas (atlanto-occipital joint) is formed by two paired structures, each pair consisting of the occipital condyle and the superior facet of the atlas. The articulating surfaces are oval, sometimes showing a beanlike configuration. The upper surface of the condyles is convex whereas the surface of the superior facets of the atlas is concave. The frontal axial angle of the joints measures on the average 124° in the adult (Fig. 8). This anatomical arrangement primarily prevents axial rotation (rotation about the Y-axis) but also side bending (rotation about the Z-axis).
The lateral aspect of the fibrous joint capsule of the atlanto-occipital joint is rigid, thereby assisting the mechanical components in restricting axial rota-

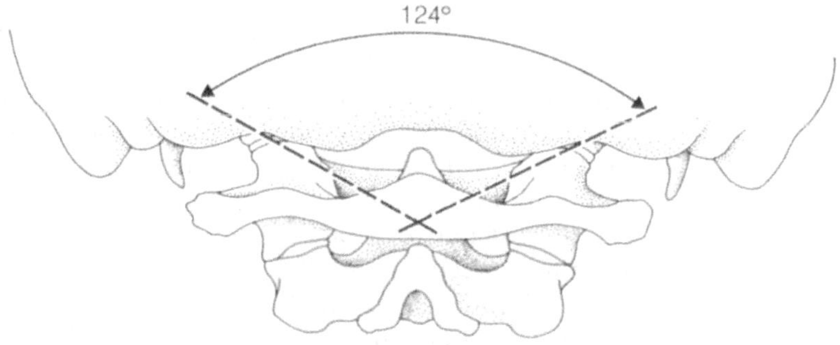

Fig. 8. Frontal axial angle of the occipital condyles; in males this angle is 124° and in females it is 127° (after Stoff 1976). The articular surfaces are in gray color

tion and sidebending. The greatest range of motion in the atlantooccipital joint is thus only possible about the X-axis, allowing primarily "inclination-reclination" motion.

The principal function of the apical alar ligaments is to secure sidebending and rotation, and indeed, in England the alar ligaments are sometimes known as the "check" ligaments.

In describing the individual motions possible in the atlanto-occipital joint, it was felt that the terms flexion and extension were inappropriate since these terms should be applied only when referring to movements about the x-axis in the entire spine. Instead, the terms incliniation and reclination were chosen specifically for the atlanto-occipital and atlanto-axial joints.

There is no doubt that the principal movement of this joint is flexion and extension (x-axis) but as to precise measurements of inclination and reclination it became clear that there exists a wide division between various countries and various authorities. (Maigne: 20°, Fielding: 10°–30°).

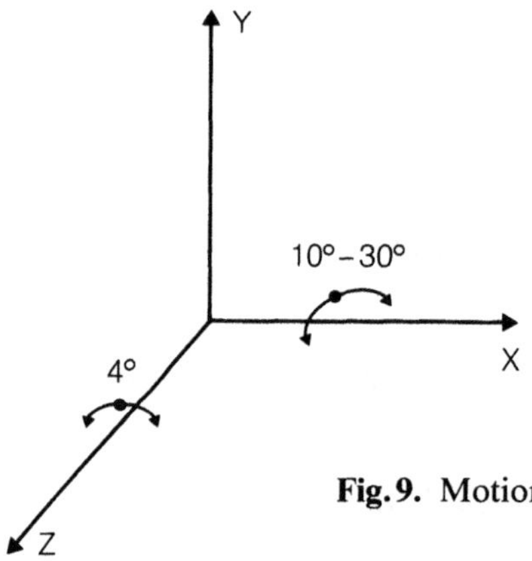

Fig. 9. Motions seen in the C0–C1 spinal segment

While no one doubted that sidebending of approximately 4° can take place at this joint (Z-axis), the question as to whether there is axial rotation (rotation about the Y-axis) provoked considerable discussion (Fig. 9). The German and Swiss schools especially feel that joint play in a rotatory sense does exist. They assess this in the "springing test." In contrast to these clinical experiences, biomechanical findings reported by Fielding, Penning, White, and Panjabi do not find any rotation in the upper cervical spinal joint (C0–C1). In the clinical setting, joint play in these joints is tested.

It is possible that, in contrast to isolated biomechanical examinations, the intact soft tissues, including cartilage of the joint surfaces, allow joint play in the living human being. CT (computed tomography) examination of this region may provide further answers to these controversial questions.

3.2.2 Atlanto-Axial Joint

This joint is very important in manual medicine. Motion takes place in four articular spaces, one of which is designated the bursa atlantodentalis; this is the space between the transverse ligament of the atlas and the dens of the axis. The transverse ligament of the atlas and the bursa atlantodentalis restrict rotation about the X-axis (flexion-extension) while it allows rotation about the Y-axis (axial rotation).
The joint surfaces are usually round, sometimes triangular and covered with cartilage of 1.4–3.2 mm thickness. The articular surfaces of the axis are convex, and those of the atlas relatively flat causing an anterior and posterior gap. The joint capsule is wide and flabby, and from the medial wall a cuneiform synovial fold reaches into the articular space (meniscoid). Sidebending between the atlas and axis is only possible with simultaneous rotation about the axis. This is also known as "forced rotation" which is mainly the result of the physiological function of the alar ligaments (Fig. 10). Undoubtedly, axial rotation is the major motion of the atlanto-axial joint. The range of motion to either side is normally 40°–50° and corresponds to a value of about half of the total cervical spine rotation.

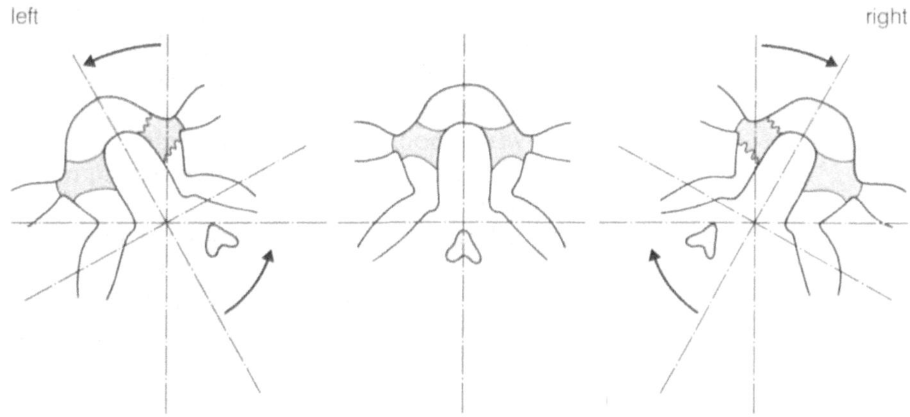

Fig. 10. Diagrammatic representation of forced rotation in the axis during sidebending of the head/cervical spine (after Dvorak and Dvorak 1983)

3.3 Diagnosis

3.3.1 Diagnostic Criteria Specific to the Cranio-Cervical Junction

All members of the group agreed that both active and passive regional examination are a definite prerequisite.

3.3.1.1 Palpation

Skin tests must be performed, the first of which is known in the English language as "skin drag." The goal of this examination is to detect any tenderness or other abnormalities discernable by palpation. Another skin test is performing the so-called "Kibler-fold," the "pincer rouler" (French school) or the "skin roll" (UK, USA). There was agreement that skin drag and skin roll are the result of a local segmental dysfunction. There exists the possibility, however, that distant changes resulting from a segmental disturbance are also responsible for such a finding (in comparison to the well known phenomenon of referred pain).

As the French school has demonstrated, the Kibler-fold in the region of the upper eyebrow may be the expression of a segmental disturbance in the suboccipital region or, using a different example, the Kibler-fold in the angle of the mandible is the result of a segmental disturbance in the C3–C4 area. This is an empirical test. The French school believes radicular irritation to be the cause of this finding, while other schools (e.g. the Swiss school) suggest a reflexogenic mechanism in the sense of a spondylogenic reflex syndrome.

3.3.1.2 Musculature

The French school, even though looking for findings such as hypertonicity and increased sensitivity in the segmental muscles does not attribute great significance to these findings. The English school, on the other hand places greater emphasis on such an evaluation but consider findings to be an indication of a segmental dysfunction.

The German school considers increased tension and pressure sensitivity found in the short suboccipital muscles (rectus capitis muscle minor, and obliquus superior muscle) to be the result of a segmental dysfunction in the atlanto-occipital joint.

The Swiss school, in addition to local and segmental muscle changes, looks for those changes due to myotendinoses in refelxogenically dependent muscle bundles.

Every school, with the exception of the French, determined in the functional examination whether shortening of the postural muscles or weakening of the phasic musculature is present in individual muscle groups. This examination is of great value and significance and dictates directly the therapeutic approach.

3.3.1.3 Apophyseal Joints

The French school concentrates on those apophyseal joints that exhibit pain attributing such findings to a segmental dysfunction.

The other schools, in particular the Swiss school, concentrate not only on segmental zones of irritation over the apophyseal joints but include also those in connective tissue regions overlying distal bony structures such as transverse and spinous processes.

The American school defines these soft tissue changes with the term "tender points," while in Germany it is known as "segmental point."

The Swiss school employs provocative testing in which there is forced motion towards the pathological barrier. An increase in painfulness at a zone of irritation is an indication of the spatial mal-positioning of the spinal segment. Both in the American and the Swiss schools the therapeutic approach, which is in the painfree direction, is based on the results obtained with the provocative tests. Treatment is into a direction which leads to decreased pain perception in the zone of irritation.

3.3.1.4 Motion Testing

C0–C1:

F: Passive inclination and reclination. The examiner concentrates on whether pain and/or restricted motion become apparent.

UK: No specific test.

AUS: The patient is supine, and one performs ballottement by compressing the head towards the atlas. An evaluation of side-to-side movement (left to right) is not possible.

FRG: With the patient in either the supine or the sitting position, joint play and end rotation between the atlas and the angle of the mandible are examined.

USA: With the patient supine, lateral gliding is examined (translatory side-to-side movement in incliniation and recliniation).

SWI: The patient is usually examined in the sitting, seldom the supine position. Of interest are joint play and end rotation between atlas and the angle to the mandible.

C1–C2:

F: Assessed are passive rotation, sidebending to the opposite side and reclination with the patient in the supine position. The examiner also takes into account any pain or diminished range of motion.

UK: No specific test.

AUS: No specific test. Rotation, inclination-reclination and sidebending movements are all tested separately.

FRG: With the patient either sitting or supine the neck is passively flexed as to fix C2, then rotation is evaluated.

SWI: With the patient sitting, maximum flexion in the cervical spine is introduced until C2 is fixed; rotational movements are examined.

C2-C3:

F: The patient is in the supine position. Passive rotation, sidebending to the same side as well as extension are evaluated. One is additionally interested whether pain is present or whether an altered range of motion is noted.

UK: No specific test.

AUS: No specific test.

FRG: The patient can be in either the sitting or the supine position: evaluated are passive sidebending of C2 with C3 being fixed (joint play).

USA:
a) With the patient supine, passive rotation and sidebending are evaluated.
b) Patient supine, passive lateral translation test.
c) Patient supine, evaluation of the motion of the posterior transverse process by introducing flexion-extension.

SWI: C1–C2 is brough to its barrier by maximal flexion, and rotation is introduced to C2–C3 while the joints distal to that are fixed through the ligaments.

3.3.2 Soft Tissue Examination

Spinal Area: C2–C7
Type of Examination: Skin palpation
Diagnostic Usefulness: Moderate: SWI
None: F, UK, AUS, FRG, USA
Procedure: The index and middle fingers evaluate superficially the skin texture, skin moisture and temperature (Figs. 11 and 12).

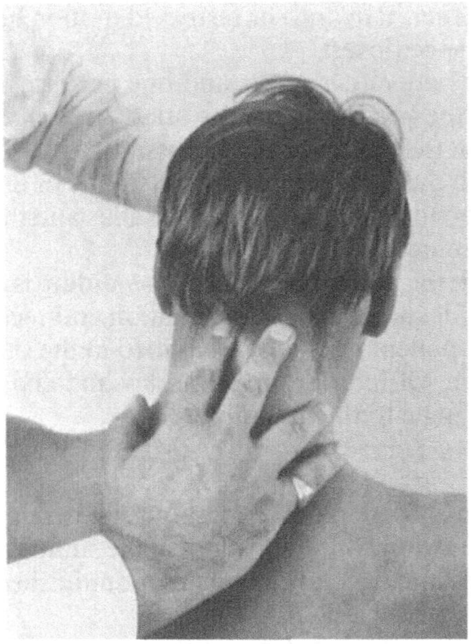
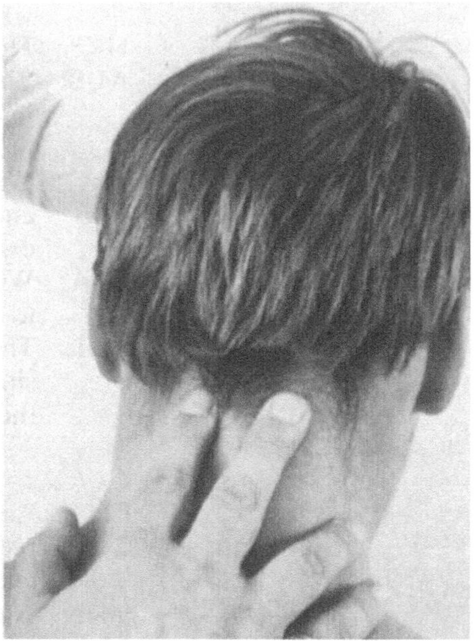

Fig. 11 **Fig. 12**

Spinal Area: C1–C2
Type of Examination: Evaluation of the subcutaneous tissue
Diagnostic Usefulness: Moderate: FRG, UK, AUS, USA, SWI
Procedure: The thumb and index finger grasp the paravertebral skin and then slide from inferior to superior ("Kibler-fold", "pincer rouler", skin rolling). This examination evaluates the ease of displacement of both skin and subcutaneous tissue, the skin's thickness and pain manifestations (Fig. 13).

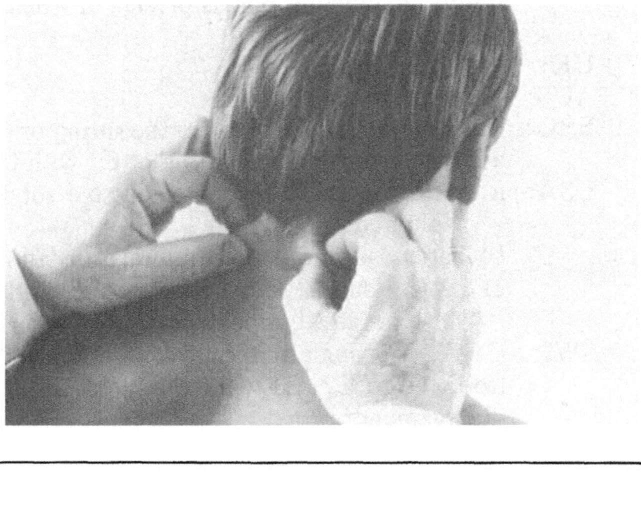

Fig. 13

Spinal Area: C2–C3

Type of Examination: Palpation of the supraorbital subcutaneous tissue

Diagnostic Usefulness: Great: F, UK.
Moderate: FRG, SWI

Procedure: With thumb and index finger a skin fold in the region of the eyebrow is formed. Sliding superiorly and inferiorly, ease of displacement and pain manifestation are evaluated (Fig. 14).

Remarks: When the fold is thickened or presents with tenderness a disturbance in segments C2–C3–C4 is often related.

Spinal Area: C2–C3

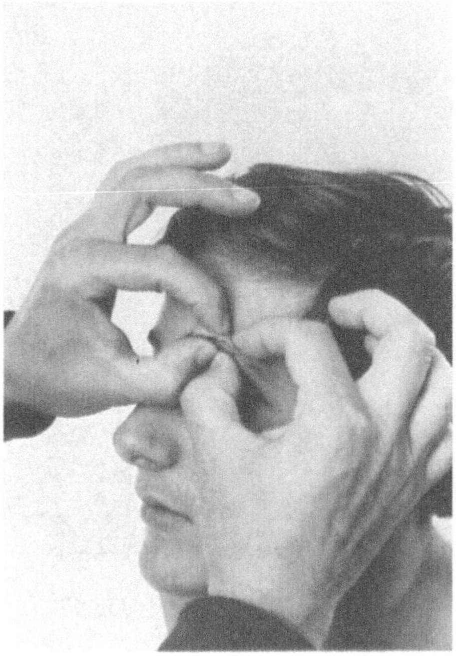

Fig. 14

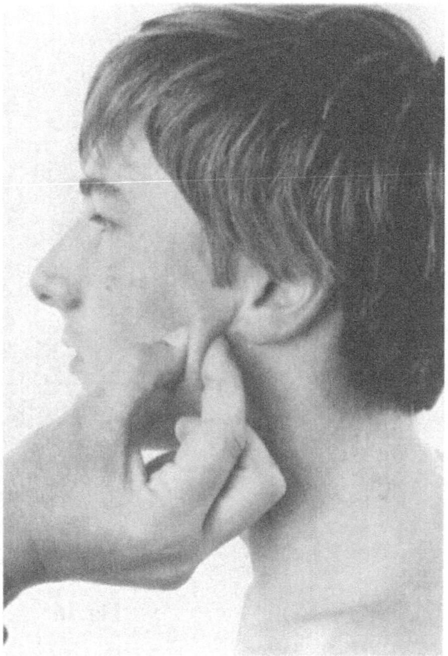

Fig. 15

Type of Examination: Skin rolling at the angle of the mandible ("pincer rouler").

Diagnostic Usefulness: Great: F
Moderate: UK
None: SWI

Procedure: One forms a skin fold between thumb and index finger in the region of the angle of the mandible. The ease of displacement of the subcutaneous tissue, skin turgor and painfulness are evaluated (Fig. 15).

Remarks: The increase in tenderness and/or turgor is related to a disturbance in the motor unit C2–C3.

Spinal Area: C2–C3
Type of Examination: Evaluation of the parietal subcutaneous tissue ("Signe de shampoo")
Diagnostic Usefulness: Great: F
Moderate: SWI
Procedure: The palpating fingers are placed over the parietal region and the skin is displaced from and to the median line. The ease of displacement or palpatory tenderness are evaluated (Fig. 16).

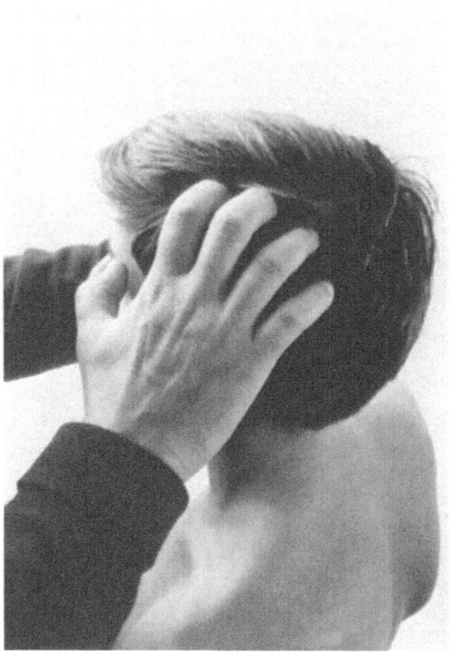

Fig. 16

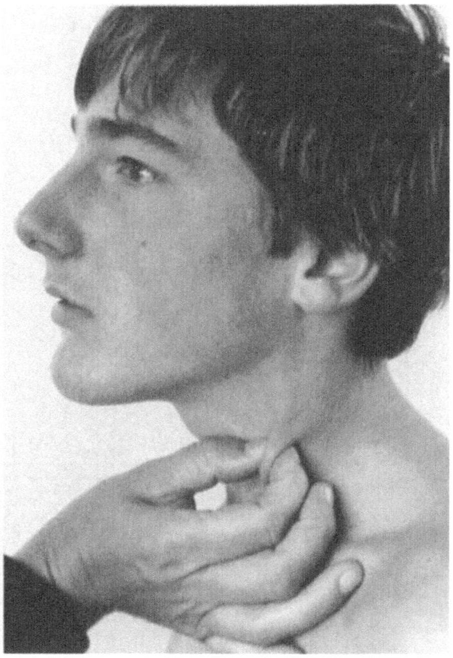

Fig. 17

Spinal Area: C3–C4
Type of Examination: Skin rolling ("Pincer rouler") in the neck region.
Diagnostic Usefulness: Great: F
Procedure: A skin fold between the thumb and index finger is formed at the neck. One evaluates the ease of displacement, skin consistency, or any pain that may be reported by the patient (Fig. 17).
Remarks: Increased painfulness as well as diminished ease of displacement are encountered with functional disturbances at the C3–C4 segment.

Spinal Area: C2–C3
Type of Examination: Evaluation of the hypoasthesic zones at the lateral aspect of the neck.
Diagnostic Usefulness: Moderate: FRG, AUS, SWI
Procedure: With a ballpoint pen constant pressure is exerted on the apophyseal joint C2–C3. The patient is asked to report the presence of pain and the radiation thereof. Pain is often found at the lateral aspect of the neck.
Remarks: When pressure on the apophyseal joint of C2–C3 elicits a hyperasthesia-zone, a dysfunction in this segment is probably present.

Spinal Area: C0–C3
Type of Examination: Palpation of the suboccipital musculature
Diagnostic Usefulness: Great: USA, AUS, UK
Moderate: SWI, F, FRG
Procedure: The patient sitting upright, rests the head against the thorax of the examiner, who stands behind the patient. The suboccipital musculature is palpated with both hands from a medio-lateral direction (Fig. 18). One is interested in increased tone, increased plasticity and increased tenderness when palpating the musculature transversely.
Remarks: In the process of this transverse palpation, it is important to be able to differentiate the individual muscle bundles so as to correctly correlate the individual painful myotendinoses with the appropriate anatomical structures.

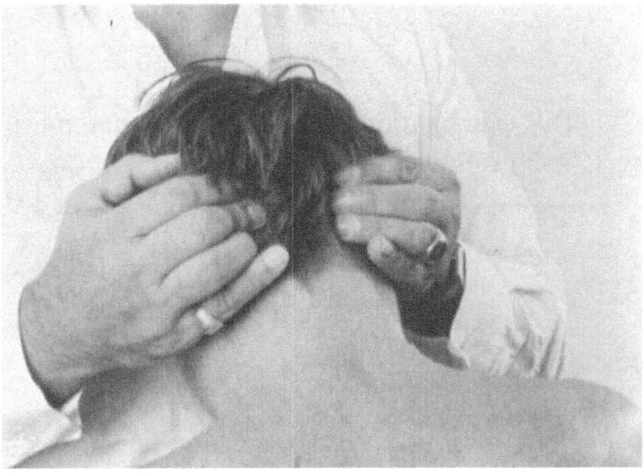

Fig. 18

Spinal Area: Craniocervical junction
Type of Examination: Examination of muscles inserting at the occiput.
Diagnostic Usefulness: Moderate: SWI, UK, FRG, F, USA, AUS
Procedure: The upright sitting patient rests his head against the examiner's thorax. The fingers palpate the muscular tendinous fibers inferiorly and follow them upwards to their respective insertions at the occiput (Fig. 19). The purpose of this procedure is to detect any changes in consistency and any painful area (tendinoses).

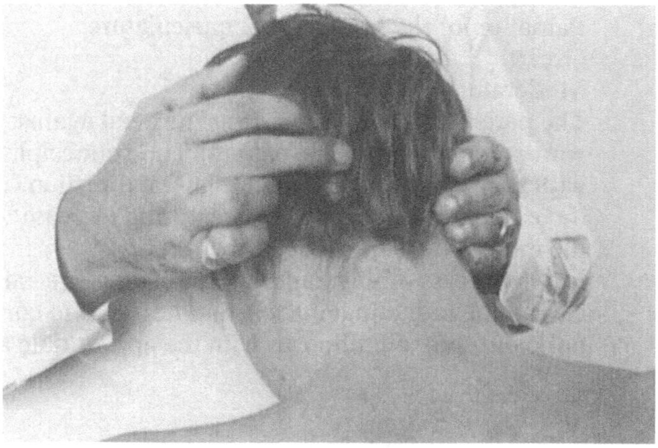

Fig. 19

Remarks: This examination requires precise anatomical knowledge of the muscles attaching at the occiput (Fig. 20).

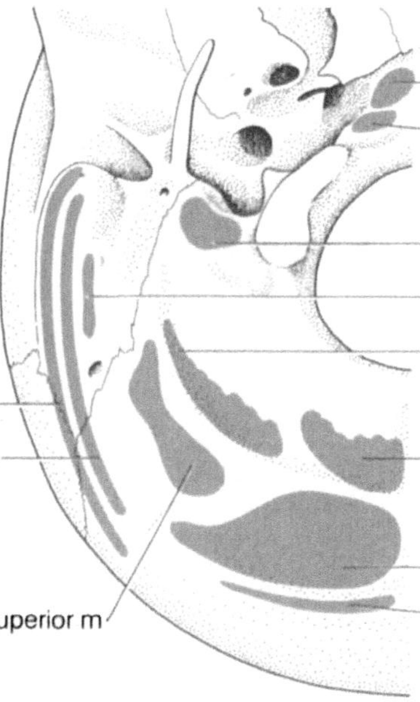

Fig. 20. Muscle attechments at the occipat. (After Dvorak and Dvorak 1983)

Spinal Area: C0–C1

Type of Examination: Palpatory examination of the superior oblique muscle and the rectus capitis posterior minor muscle.

Diagnostic Usefulness: Great: FRG
Moderate: SWI

Procedure: The patient is in the sitting position with the head slightly extended backward. The middle finger palpates first the transverse process of the atlas and then the tendon attachment of the superior oblique muscle by going from superior to inferior (Fig. 21). It is important to evaluate the tendon along its fiber direction which is in contrast to the muscle belly, where palpation is perpendicular.

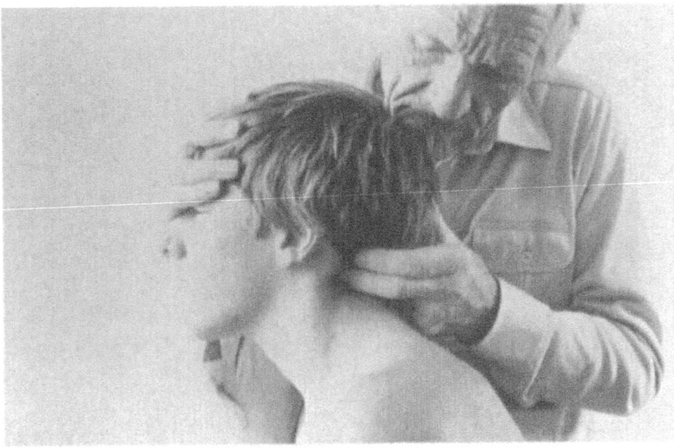

Fig. 21

Spinal Area: C1–C2

Type of Examination: Palpation of the inferior obliquus capitis muscle and the rectus capitis posterior major muscle.

Diagnostic Usefulness: Great: FRG
Moderate: SWI

Procedure: The head of the sitting patient is held passively in a slightly extended position. The operator's middle finger palpates the transverse process of the atlas, and then follows the inserting tendon of the obliquus inferior muscle from inferior to superior (Fig. 22). The index finger then palpates the spinous process of the atlas, and the origin-tendon of the rectus capitis posterior major muscle is located by moving from supero-laterally to medio-inferiorly arriving at the spinous process of C2. One tries to elicit painful myotendinoses or tension changes in the individual muscles.

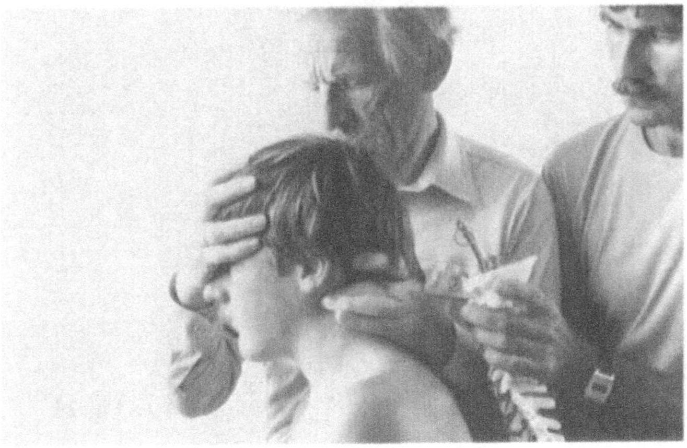

Fig. 22

Spinal Area: C2–C3

Type of Examination: Palpation of the neck muscles.

Diagnostic Usefulness: Moderate: FRG, SWI

Procedure: With the patient sitting, the superior edge of thc hyoid bone is palpated with both thumbs moving from laterally to medially (Fig. 23).
The tension of the individual muscles and any tenderness at the individual muscle insertions are evaluated (Fig. 24).

Remarks: This examination is of great importance in patients who present with dysphagia of unknown origin, which may be caused by spondylogenic disturbances and may be related to the C2–C3 segment.

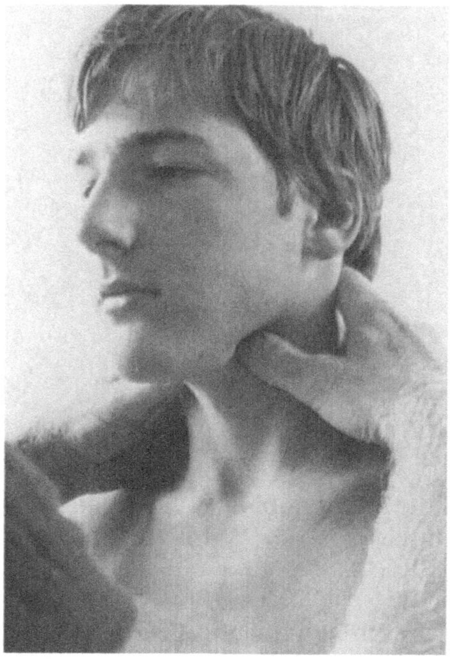

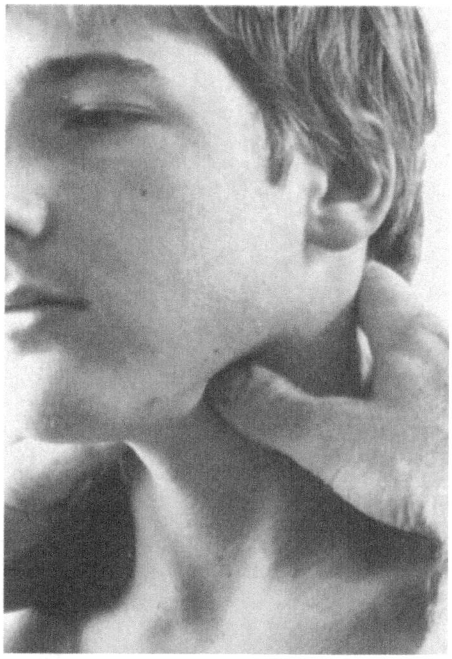

Fig. 23 Fig. 24

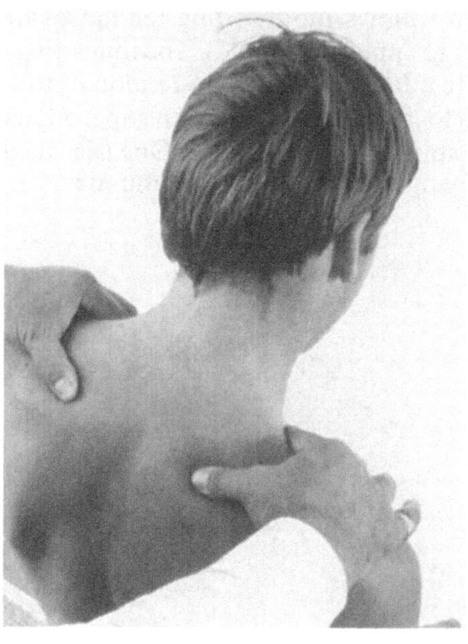

Fig. 25

Spinal Area: C1–C4
Type of Examination: Palpation of the levator scapulae muscle.
Diagnostic Usefulness: Great: SWI, FRG
Moderate: UK, AUS

Procedure: The levator scapulae muscle arises by four fasciculi from the transverse processes of the first four cervical vertebrae. The first tendon, which is also the strongest, folds around the transverse process of the atlas latero-anteriorly. The muscle inserts at the medial border of the scapula between the superior angle and the base of the spine of the scapula. While one is not able to use palpation to differentiate between the origins of this muscle the insertion-tendinosis, in contrast, located at the medial border of the scapula can be easily palpated. Due to the steep angle at which the muscle inserts, the palpatory direction is from superior (Fig. 25).

Spinal Area: C2–C3
Type of Examination: Palpation of the apophyseal joints
Diagnostic Usefulness: Great: FRG, AUS, F, UK, USA, SWI
Procedure: The patient is in the supine position, and his head is slightly flexed (Fig. 26). The Swiss school, in contrast, prefers the patient sitting (Fig. 27). The fingers palpate the strong semispinalis capitis muscle first and then reach a muscular groove which is formed deeply between the semispinalis capitis muscle and the longissimus capitis muscle. The first prominent bony mass that is encountered under the occiput is the apophyseal joint C2–C3. Evaluated are quality of motion, local edematous changes and especially areas that become painful when pressure is applied.

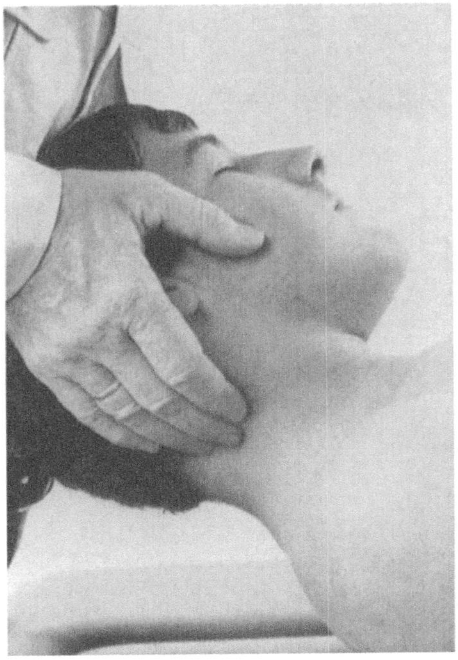

Fig. 26

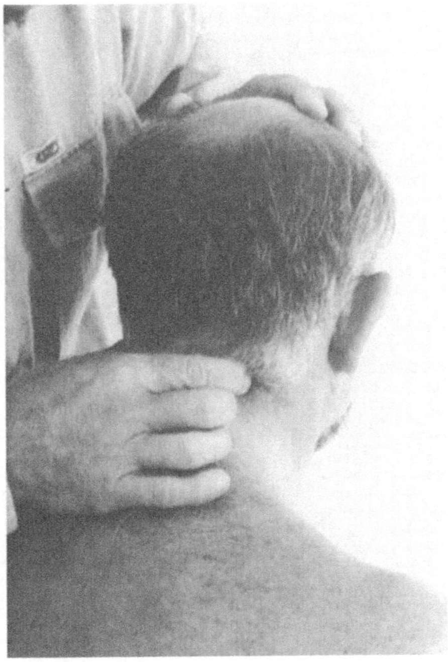

Fig. 27

Spinal Area:	C0–C1
Type of Examination:	Segmental zone of irritation at the occiput
Diagnostic Usefulness:	Great: SWI, F
Procedure:	Emperically one can find two zones of irritation at the occiput which are related to the position of the occiput and the atlas. The zone of irritation that correlates to the occiput lies lateral and upper to the superior end of the mastoid notch (the non-muscular bony portion between the splenius capitis muscle and obliquus capitis superior muscle (Figs. 28, 29). The zone of irritation that relates to the atlas lies medial and inferior to the superior end of the mastoid notch. A dysfunction affecting the atlanto-occipital joint often presents with these zones of irritation. Provocative testing, however, is necessary to differentiate between these zones of irritation and the surrounding myotendinoses of the suboccipital musculature.
Remarks:	Upon provocative testing, the zones of irritation in the cervical spine react with decreased painfulness and noticeable tissue changes. The finding of decreased tenderness indicates the therapeutic direction applicable for that individual segment.

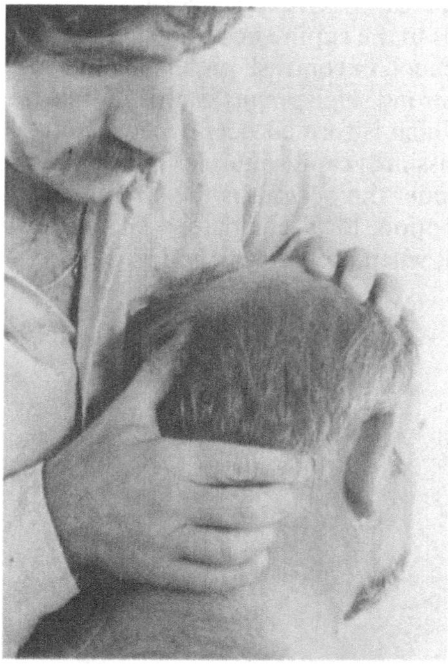

Fig. 28

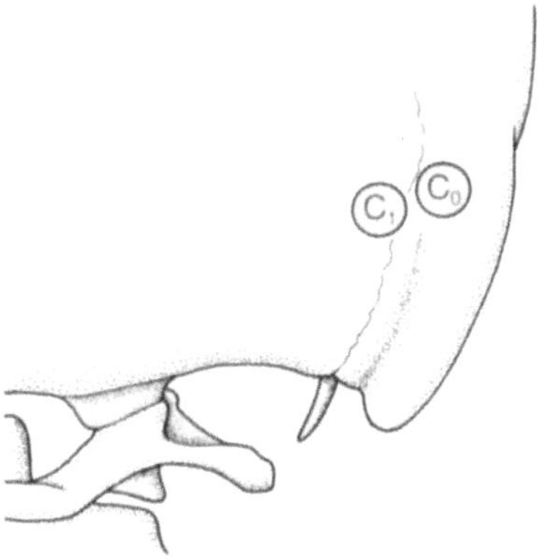

Fig. 29. Zone of irritation C0–C1 located at the occiput (Dvorak and Dvorak 1983)

3.3.3 Motion Testing

Spinal Area: Entire cervical spine

Type of Examination: Testing for rotation-sidebending and translatory flexion-extension movements

Diagnostic Usefulness: Great: AUS
Moderate: SWI

Procedure: With the patient supine and his head slightly flexed, the operator's fingers palpate through the muscular groove formed by the semispinalis capitis and longissimus capitis muscles as to reach the apophyseal joints bilaterally. The palm of the hand grasps the parietal region of the head introducing passive flexion and extension (Figs. 30, 31), axial rotation and translatory sidebending. Evaluated are overall range of motion and the limits of range of motion in each individual apophyseal joint.

Remarks: It should be noted that coupling patterns are most prominent in the cervical region (axial rotation, for instance, is always coupled with sidebending).

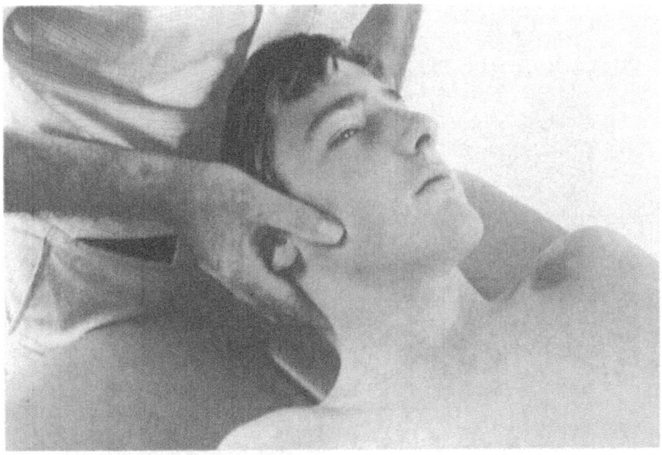

Fig. 30

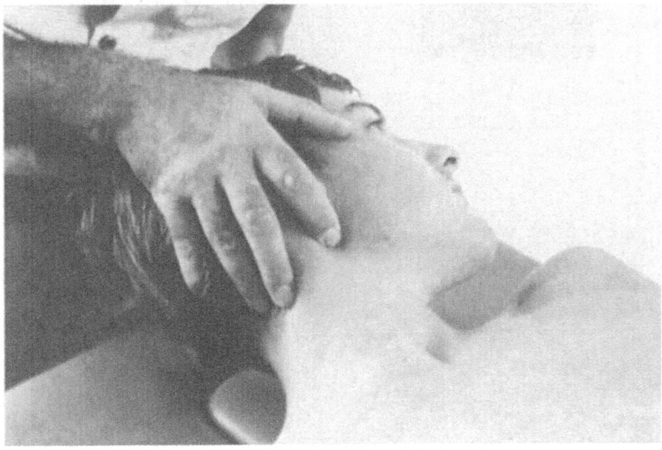

Fig. 31

Spinal Area: C0–C1

Type of Examination: Evaluation of inclination and reclination movement in the atlanto-occipital joint.

Diagnostic Usefulness: Great: F

Procedure: The head of the upright sitting patient rests on the examiner's thorax who is standing in front of the patient. The examiner's hands are placed at the temporal region with the fingers palpating the small suboccipital musculature. A passive inclination and reclination motion is introduced (Fig. 32), and the palpating fingers evaluate any changes in muscle tone and the appearance of pain in the region of the suboccipital musculature. The appearance of pain especially is considered to be related to a segmental dysfunction in the atlanto-occipital joint.

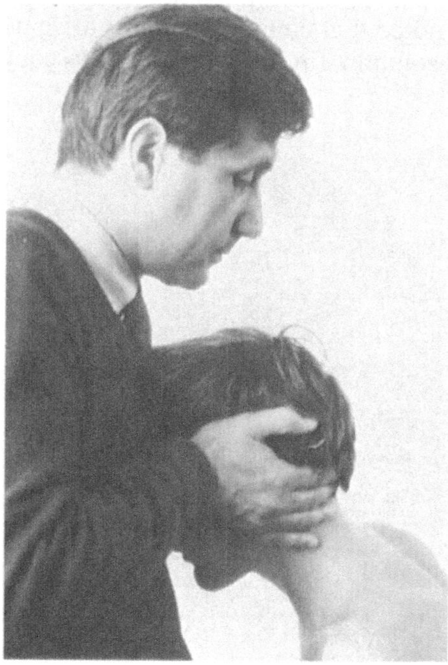

Fig. 32

Spinal Area: C0–C1
Type of Examination: Ballottement test
Diagnostic Usefulness: Great: AUS
Procedure: The patient is supine. In a vise-like manner, the examiner's thumbs and index fingers grasp the occiput. The palm of the hand supports the occiput. The operator's other hand is placed on the patient's vortex of the head for stabilization (Fig. 33). With his supporting hand under the occiput the examiner introduces traction of the head while he palpates joint play in this area.
Remarks: This examination does not provide information as to which side is involved.

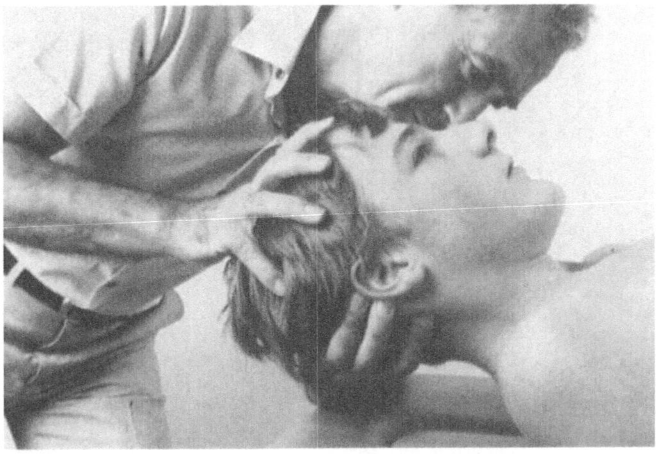

Fig. 33

Spinal Area: C0–C1
Type of Examination: Evaluation of rotation motion in the atlanto-occipital joint
Diagnostic Usefulness: Great: FRG, SWI
Procedure: The examiner palpates with his middle finger the transverse process at the atlas of the patient, who is seated. The other hand is placed over the temporal region and introduces maximum passive rotation of the head (Fig. 34). Having reached the barrier, a springing type of rotational motion is introduced and with the palpating middle finger joint play of the atlas is evaluated.

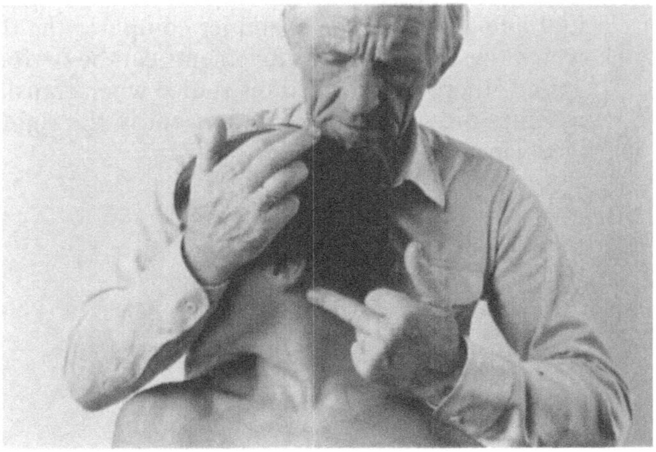

Fig. 34

Spinal Area: C0–C1
Type of Examination: Evaluation for sidebending
Diagnostic Usefulness: Great: FRG
Procedure: The patient is supine with the head maximally flexed. In this position one introduces passive sidebending so as to evaluate joint play at the barriers (Fig. 35).

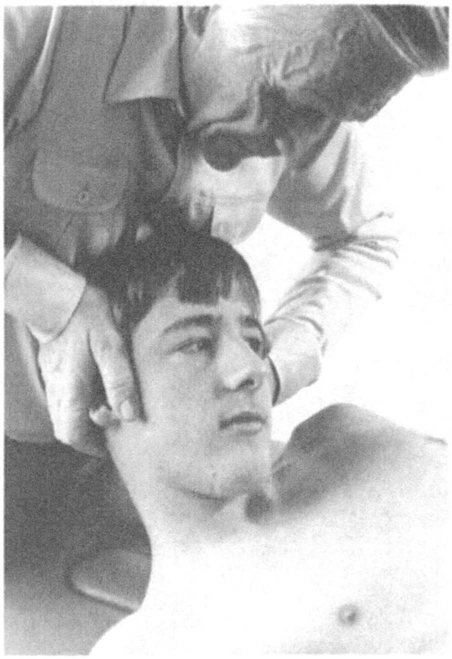

Fig. 35

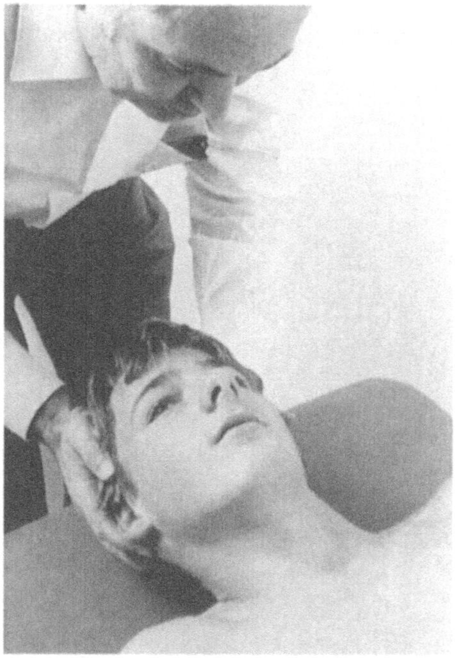

Fig. 36

Spinal Area: C0–C1
Type of Examination: Evaluation of translatory gliding motion in the atlanto-occipital joint
Diagnostic Usefulness: Great: USA
Procedure: With the patient supine, the examiner palpates the occipital condyles (postero-lateral condyle region). The hands are placed over the temporal region of the head and introduce translatory motion from left to right, both with the head flexed and extended. The head, however, remains fixed in the mid-sagittal line (Fig. 36). The examiner compares the difference in resistance with which these translatory movements can be performed (side to side comparison). If there is increased resistance when translating from right to left, one assumes a dysfunction to be present in the right atlanto-occipital joint and vice-versa.

Spinal Area: C1–C2
Type of Examination: Evaluation of coupling patterns (rotation-sidebending)
Diagnostic usefulness: Great: F
Procedure: With the patient supine, the examiner's hands are placed over the temporal region allowing the index fingers to palpate the suboccipital area. The head is first extended and then rotated and sidebent (Fig. 37). If pain is elicited during this maneuver, one assumes that a dysfunction is present in the atlanto-axial joint.

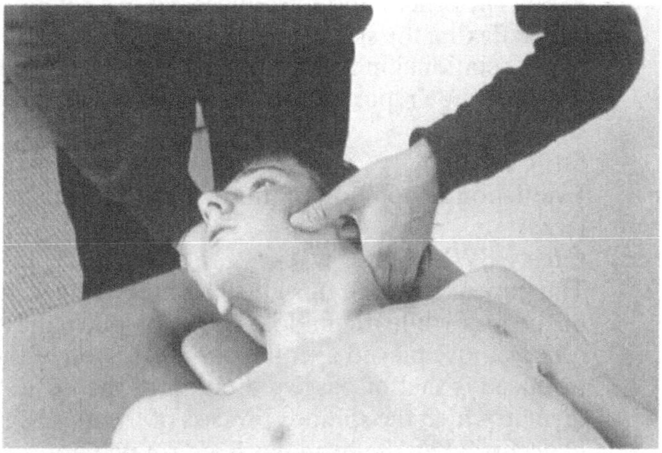

Fig. 37

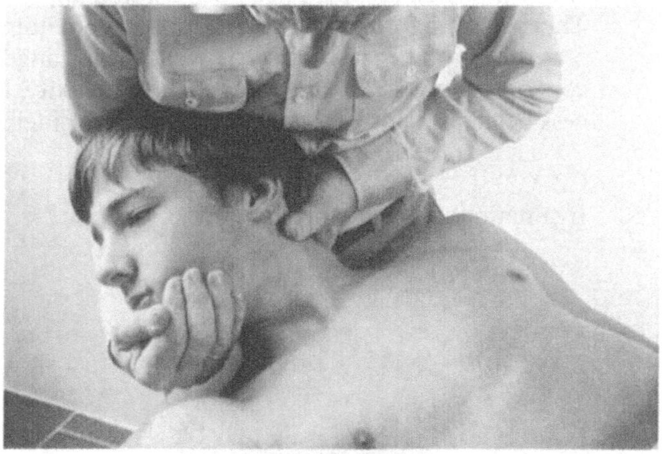

Fig. 38

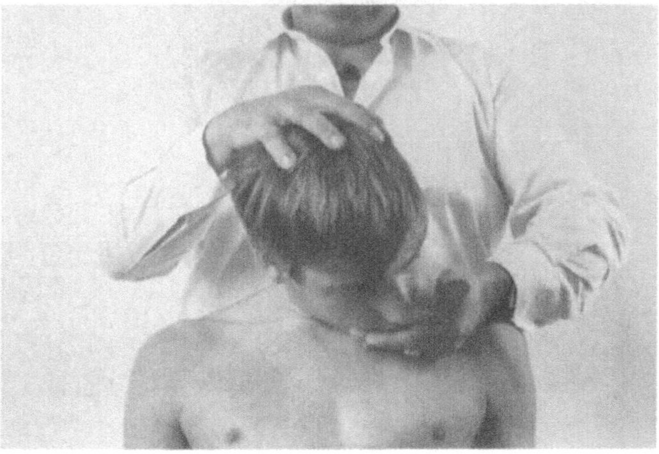

Fig. 39

Spinal area: C1–C2
Type of Examination: Evaluation of rotation motion with the cervical spine in maximal flexion
Diagnostic Usefulness: Great: FRG, SWI
Procedure: *FRG:* with the patient supine, the examiner stabilizes with one hand the axis from both sides while the other hand cradles the patient's chin. After having introduced maximum flexion in the cervical spine passive rotation is introduced (Fig. 38).
SWI: the patient is in a sitting, slightly slouched position. The cervical spine is flexed passively to the barrier, so the chin comes to rest at the patient's chest. The other hand introduces passive rotation (Fig. 39).
Remarks: When flexing the spine maximally the segments below C2 cannot participate in the rotational movement so that rotation occurs only then in C1–C2. The average value reported for this motion is 45° to either side.

Spinal Area: C1–C2
Type of Examination: Evaluation of rotation motion of the axis (axial rotation and coupling patterns)
Diagnostic Usefulness: Great: SWI
Procedure: The patient is sitting upright. The index finger palpates the spinous process of the axis while the middle finger palpates the spinous process of C3. The other hand is placed over the parietal region of the head. The first motion introduced is that of passive rotation of the head. One tries to detect the moment at which the spinous process of the axis begins to move, which normally occurs when the head has been rotated approximately 20° (Fig. 40).
Then, starting from a neutral position, sidebending is introduced. One evaluates the character of motion as well as the range of motion of spinous process of the axis in the direction of the convexity. In this test, the spinous process begins to move at the moment passive sidebending is introduced.

Spinal Area: C2–C3
Type of Examination: Evaluation of translatory motion

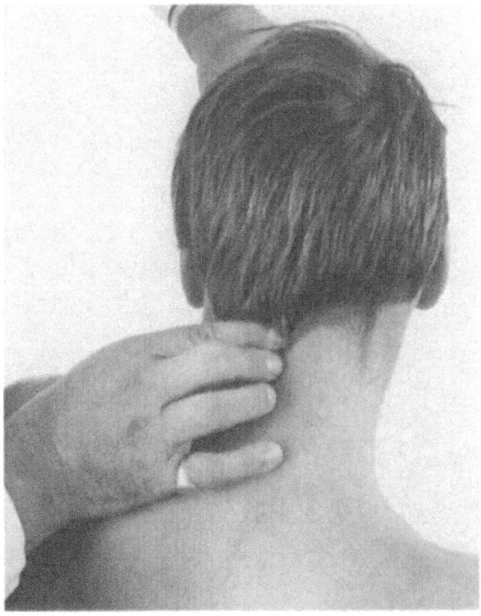

Fig. 40

Diagnostic Usefulness: Great: FRG, USA

Procedure: *FRG:* The patient is supine and the head is slightly flexed. The index finger palpates the transverse process of C2 and with a springing type of motion moves it medially to the barrier while the head is simultaneously sidebent. One evaluates joint play and translatory motion of C2 (Fig. 41).

USA: the patient is also supine. The operator who is positioned superior to the patient palpates the apophyseal joints of C2–C3 bilaterally. With the introduction of slight extension in the neck, C2 is translated laterally with the index finger (Fig. 42). One evaluates range of motion and joint play in the C2–C3 segment.

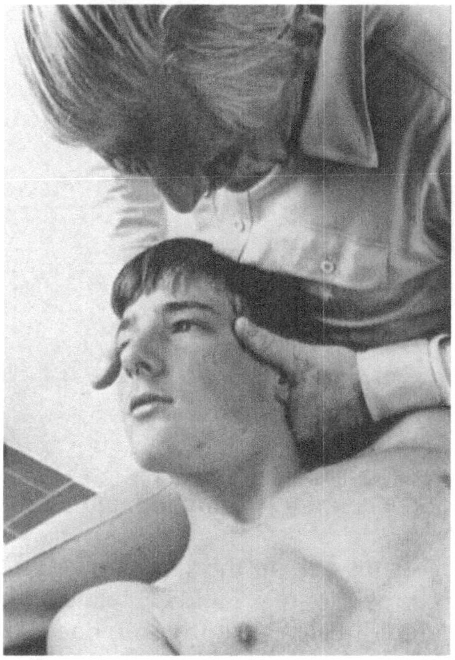

Fig. 41

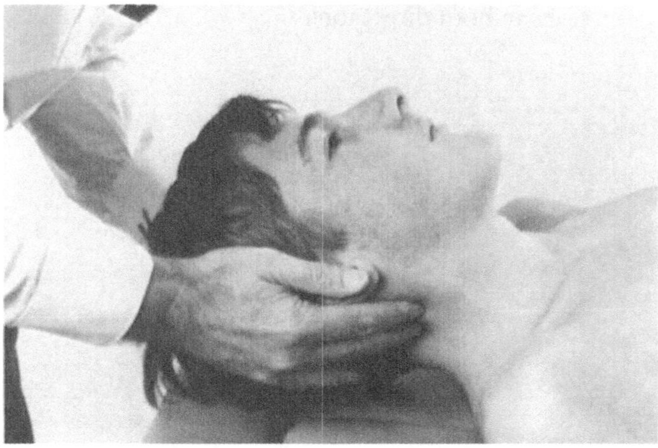

Fig. 42

Spinal Area: C2–C3
Type of Examination: Evaluation of rotation and sidebending with the head either inclined or reclined
Diagnostic Usefulness: Great: F
Procedure: The head of the supine patient is rotated passively and sidebent passively to the same side. In this position, passive inclination and reclination motion is introduced. One is interested if pain appears during this maneuver, which would indicate a segmental dysfunction in the C2–C3 segment.

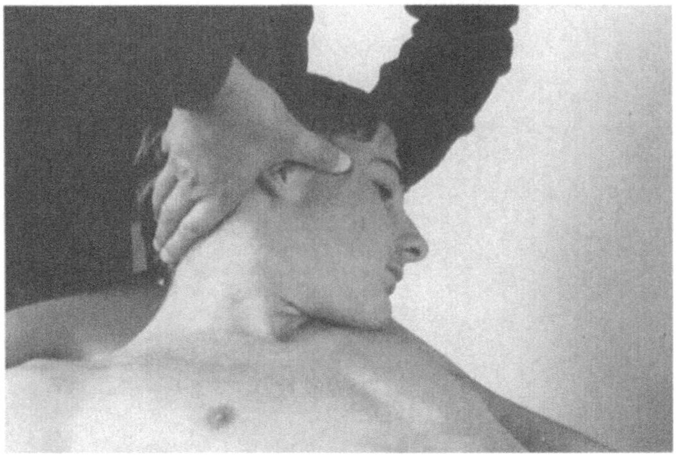

Fig. 43

Spinal Area: C2–C3
Type of Examination: Evaluation of the coupling of rotation and sidebending
Diagnostic Usefulness: Great: USA
Procedure: The operator stands behind the supine patient. Both index fingers palpate the transverse processes of C2 and C3 bilaterally, and slight extension of the head is introduced. From this position, one starts a rotation motion along with sidebending as to evaluate the extent of resistance or ease of these motions in both direct ions.

Spinal Area: C2–C3

Type of Examination: Evaluation of rotation of the head with the C1–C2 segment inclined

Diagnostic Usefulness: Great: SWI

Procedure: With the patient in the sitting position, the head is inclined passively to its barrier (the chin is drawn towards the body while the cervical spine remains extended). In this postion, passive rotation is introduced (Fig. 44). The normal values for this rotational movement range between 20° and 25°.

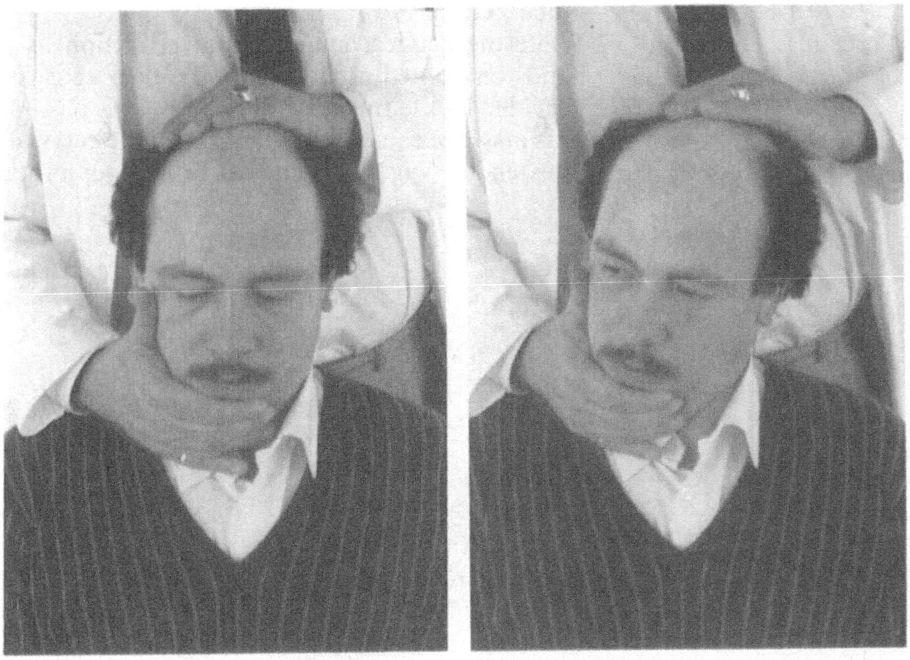

Fig. 44

3.4 Treatment

3.4.1 Soft Tissue Treatment

Type of Treatment: Traction massage
Goal: Pain reduction, and patient relaxation
Technique: Traction massage
Therapeutic Usefulness: Great: FRG, SWI, AUS, USA
None: UK
Procedure: While the cervical spine is under traction as provided by the operator's hands on the temporal region, the neck muscles undergo lateral stretch as provided by the fingertips (Fig. 45).
Remarks: This massage can be carried out with the cervical spine either flexed (Fig. 46) or extended (Fig. 47), both with or without a rotation component.

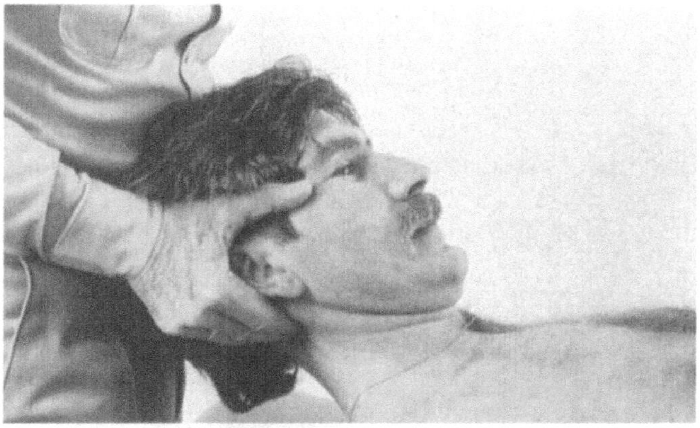

Fig. 45

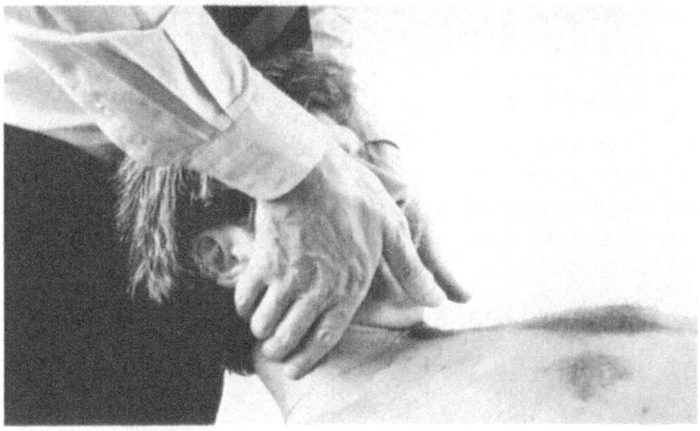

Fig. 46

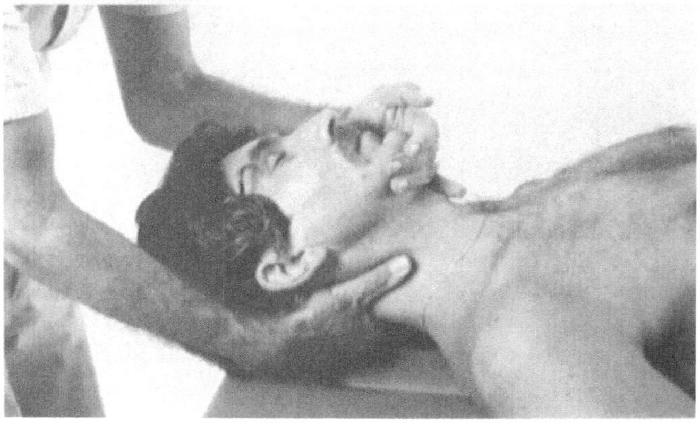

Fig. 47

3.4.2 Mobilization Without Impulse (No Thrust)

Type of treatment: Mobilization without impulse
Goal: Improvement of inclination between C0–C1
Technique: Mobilization
Therapeutic Usefulness: Great: F, UK
Procedure: The patient is supine, and the operator places his hand on the forehead and occiput (Fig. 48). With C0–C1 in the inclination (flexed) position; mobilization is applied to this area.

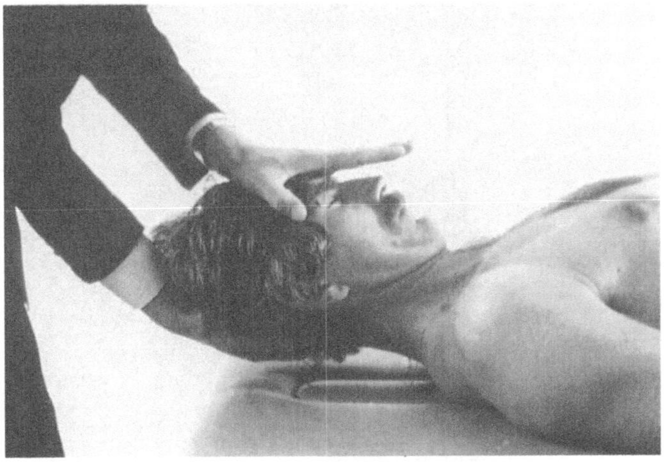

Fig. 48

Type of Treatment: Mobilization without impulse
Goal: Improvement of joint play at C0–C1
Technique: Translation mobilization
Therapeutic Usefulness: Great: AUS
Procedure: The patient is supine and his head is stabilized by the operator who places his hands over the patient's mandible and occiput (Fig. 49). Mobilization is in the lateral direction.

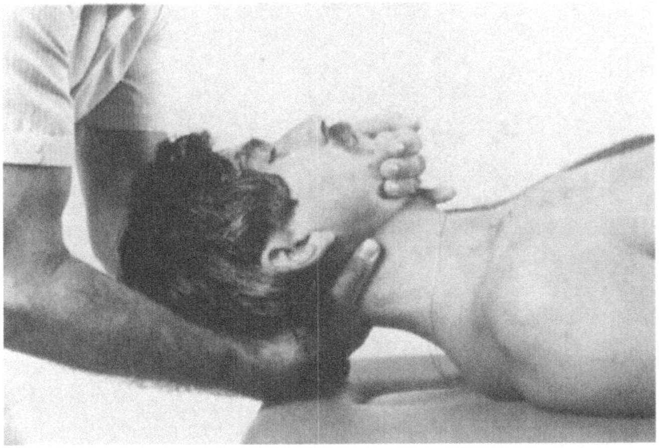

Fig. 49

Type of Treatment: Mobilization without impulse
Goal: Improvement of joint play at C0–C1 (posterior gliding)
Technique: Mobilization
Therapeutic Usefulness: Great: FRG
Procedure: The patient is supine, and with a vise-like grip the atlas is fixed. The operator's hand placed over the patient's forehead exerts posterior pressure (Figs. 50 and 51). This results in mobilization of C0–C1.

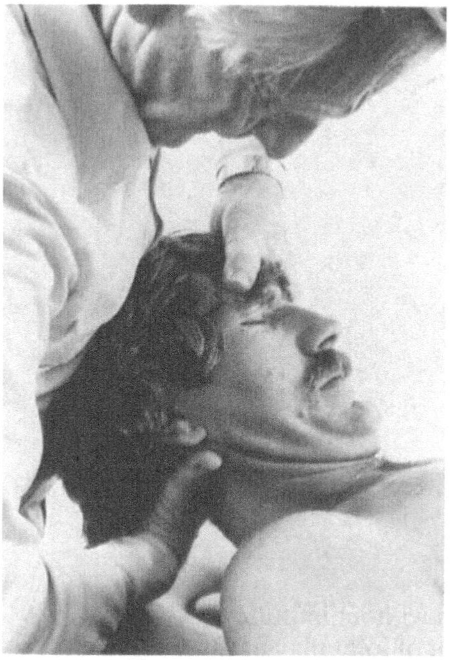

Fig. 50

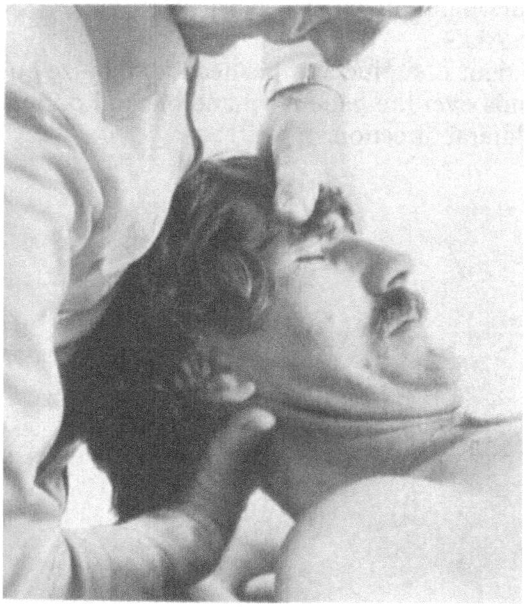

Fig. 51

Type of Treatment: Mobilization without impulse
Goal: Improvement of joint play between C0–C1 and C2–C3
Technique: Flexion and extension mobilization
Therapeutic Usefulness: Great: SWI
Procedure: The patient is sitting. The operator fixes C3 by holding its articular processes in a vise-like manner. The other hand is placed flat over the temporal region and the occiput while the head is placed against the operator's chest and forearm. Slight traction is introduced to the cervical spine (Fig. 52). Mobilization is in a posterior and anterior direction.

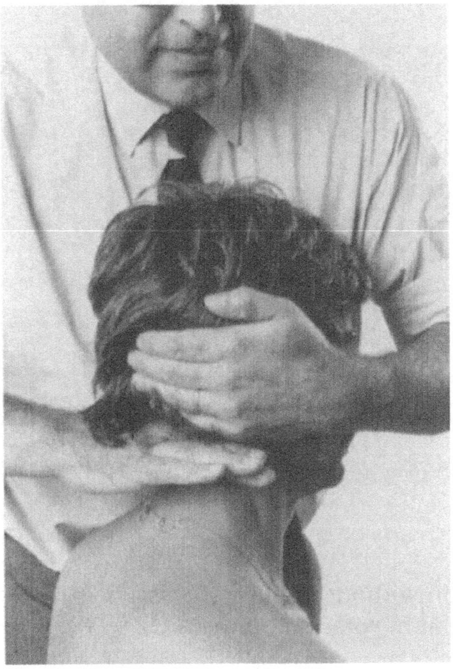

Fig. 52

Type of Treatment: Mobilization without impulse
Goal: Improvement of rotation at C1–C2
Technique: Rotation mobilization
Therapeutic Usefulness: Great: FRG
Procedure: The patient is supine. In a vise-like grip, C2 is stabilized. Passive rotation of the head is effected by the operator placing his hand over the patient's chin and resting the patient's head against his chest (Fig. 53).

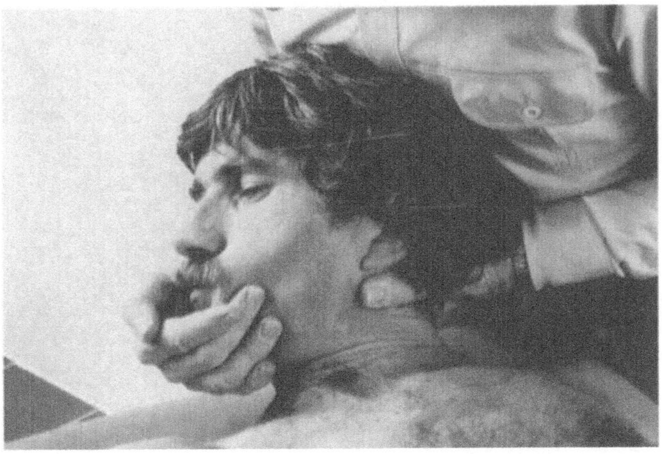

Fig. 53

Type of Treatment: Mobilization without impulse
Goal: Improvement of rotation at C1–C2
Technique: Rotation mobilization
Therapeutic Usefulness: Great: AUS
Procedure: The patient is supine. The head is stabilized with both of the operator's hands. Rotation to the cervical spine is then introduced (i.e., to the right). The proximal phalanx of the first finger palpates the right portion of the vertebral and of the atlas (Fig. 54). Right rotation mobilization is introduced by the operator's left hand.

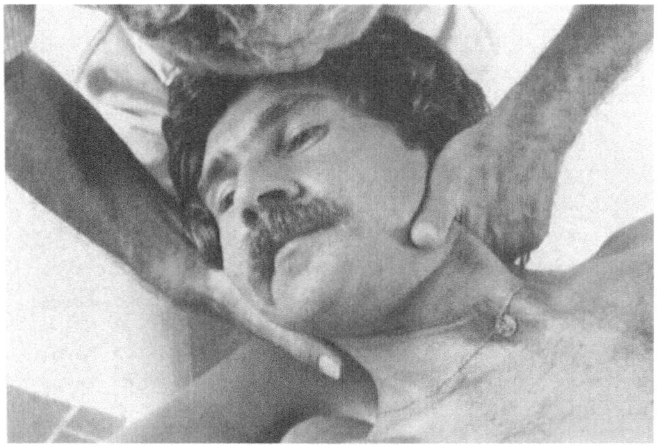

Fig. 54

Type of Treatment: Mobilization without impulse (thrust)
Goal: Improvement of rotation between C2–C3
Technique:
Therapeutic Usefulness: Great: AUS
Procedure: The operator places both hands over the temporal region and the articular pillars of C2 are palpated with both index fingers. As in this example, the cervical spine is passively rotated to the right. The rotational force is enhanced with the left index finger pressing on the articular process of C2 (Fig. 55).

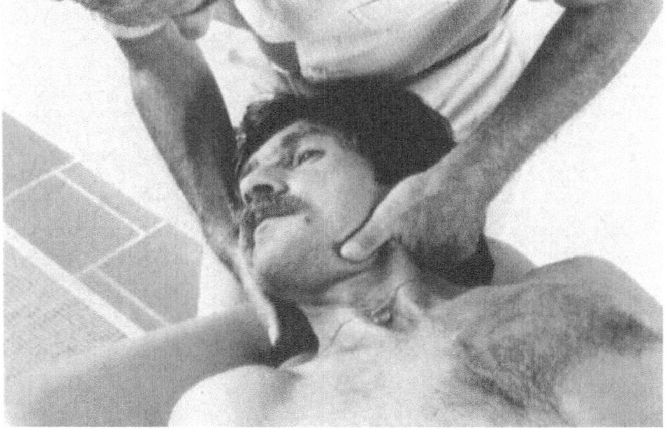

Fig. 55

3.4.3 Mobilization With Impulse (Thrust Techniques)

Type of Treatment: Mobilization with impulse
Goal: Improvement of reclination at C0–C1
Technique: Extension manipulation
Therapeutic Usefulness: Great: USA
Procedure: As in this example, the cervical spine is rotated to the left (the restricted side). The vertebrae C_0 to C_3 are extended. Sidebending to the right is introduced. The operator's index finger palpates the occiput with the right hand (Fig. 56). The impulse is towards the patient's nose.
Remarks: The same technique can be applied for the segment C2–C3.

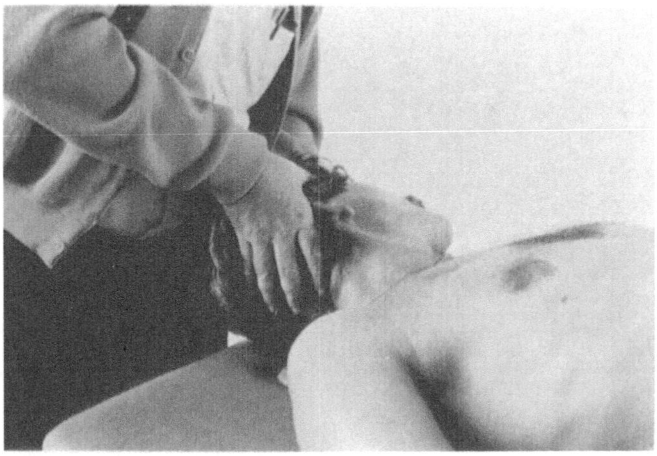

Fig. 56

Type of Treatment: Mobilization with impulse
Goal: Improvement of reclination between C0–C1
Technique: Extension manipulation
Therapeutic Usefulness: Great: AUS
Procedure: The patient is supine and his head is stabilized by the operator's thorax and right hand (in this example). The cervical spine is then rotated to one side (i.e., right) while the operator's other hand is placed in a vise-like manner around the occiput (Fig. 57).
The impulse is directed laterally to the right and superiorly.

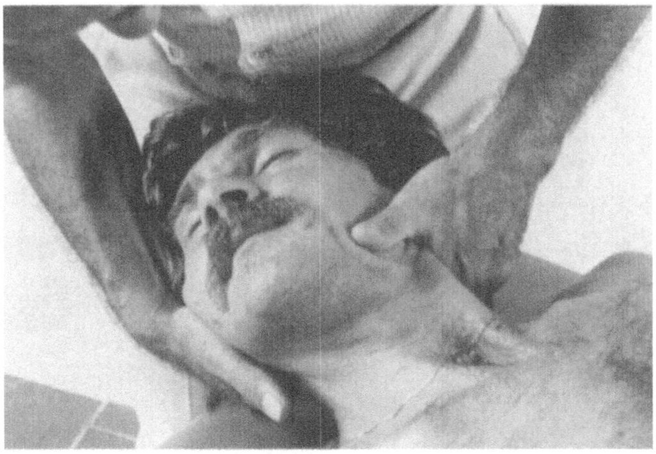

Fig. 57

Type of Treatment: Mobilization with impulse
GoalßGoal: Improvement of joint play between C0–C1
Technique: Extension manipulation
Therapeutic Usefulness: Great: SWI-CH
Procedure: The patient is sitting. The atlas is stabilized through a vise-like grip. Maximum rotation in the cervical spine is introduced to the left, for instance, in combination with reclination between C_0 and C_1 and extension down to C_3. The operator's other hand is placed over the patient's head, and the occipital and bitemporal regions are stabilized by way of the operator's thorax and hand (Fig. 58).
The impulse is directed superiorly.

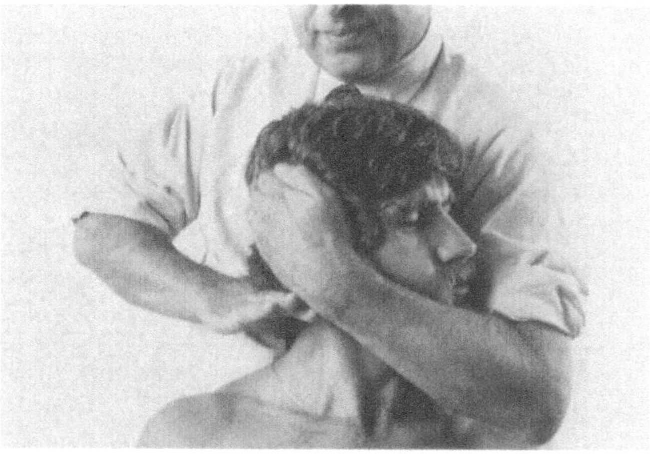

Fig. 58

Type of Treatment: Mobilization with impulse
Goal: Improvement of joint play between C0–C1
Technique: Rotation and sidebending manipulation
Therapeutic Usefulness: Great: FRG
Procedure: The patient is supine. Slight flexion and sidebending of approximately 5° to the restricted side are introduced in the cervical spine. The proximal phalanx of the second finger is placed over the mastoid process. The barrier is engaged (Fig. 59), and the impulse through the mastoid process is in a superolateral direction.

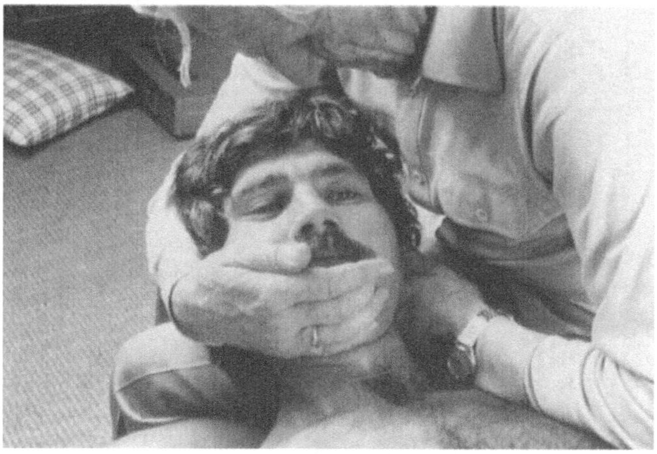

Fig. 59

Type of Treatment: Mobilization with impulse
Goal: Improvement of joint play at C1–C2
Technique: Translation manipulation
Therapeutic Usefulness: Great: FRG, AUS
Procedure: The patient is supine, and the cervical spine is flexed. C2 is fixed at the transverse processes through a vise-like grip (Figs. 60, 61).
The metacarpal joint of the index finger with of his other hand the operator provides a translatory type of impulse upon the transverse process of C1.

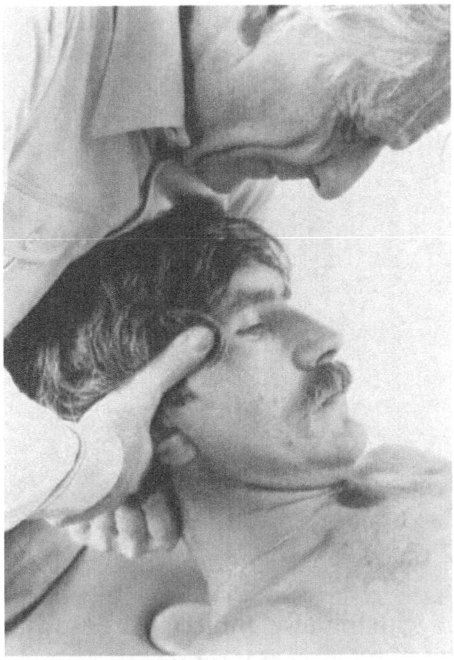
Fig. 60

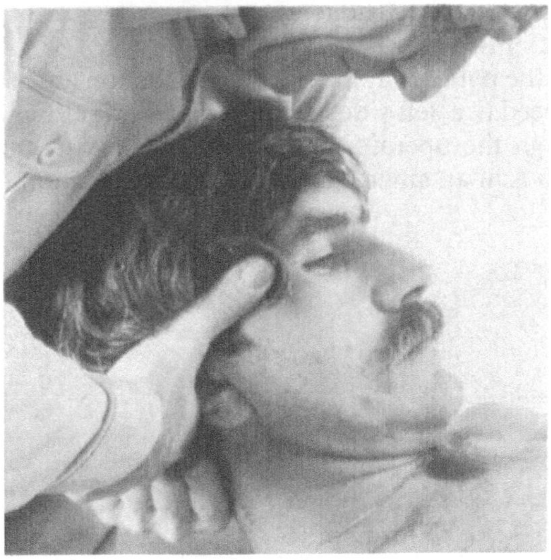
Fig. 61

Type of Treatment: Mobilization with impulse
Goal: Improvement of joint play between C0–C1
Technique: Rotation manipulation
Therapeutic Usefulness: Great: FRG
Procedure: The patient is supine, and the cervical spine is maximally flexed. As in this example, rotation is introduced to the right. The operator's proximal phalanx of the left second finger is placed over the occiput and mastoid. The patient's head is fixed at the chin by the operator's right hand and the operator's thorax (patient's occiput). The impulse is directed towards the patient's eyes (Fig. 62).

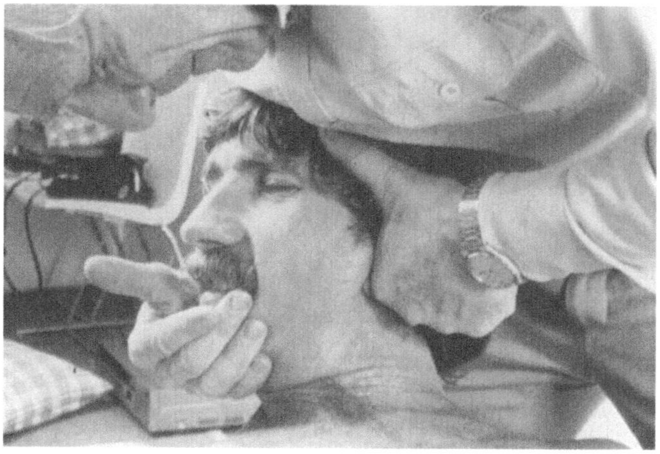

Fig. 62

Type of Treatment: Mobilization with impulse (thrust)
Goal: Improvement of rotation at C1–C2
Technique: Rotation manipulation
Therapeutic Usefulness: Great: FRG
Procedure: With the patient supine, maximum flexion and sidebending to one side is introduced (i.e. left side) in the cervical spine (Fig. 63). The impulse is effected through the operator's proximal phalanx of the index finger on the atlas which is in an antero-lateral and right direction.

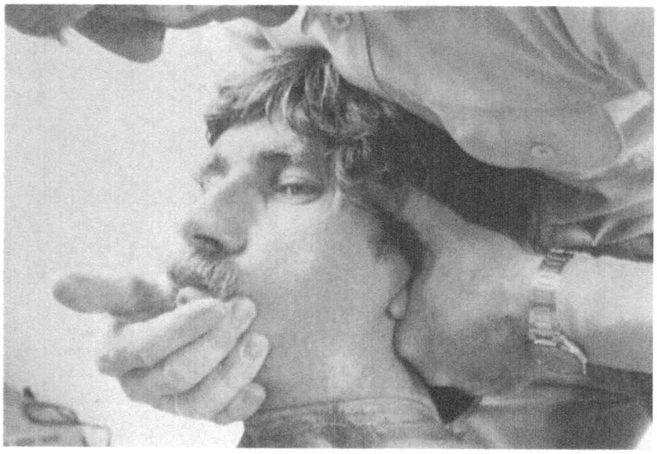

Fig. 63

Type of Treatment: Mobilization with impulse
Goal: Improvement of rotation at C1–C2
Technique: Rotation manipulation
Therapeutic Usefulness: Great: SWI
Procedure: The patient is sitting. The cervical spine is maximally sidebent to one side (e.g. left side). The patient's head is then fixed by the operator's left hand which is placed over the temporo-occipital region. The middle finger of the other hand (right) is placed over the right lateral mass of the atlas with (Fig. 64). The impulse is in direction of rotation at the atlas.

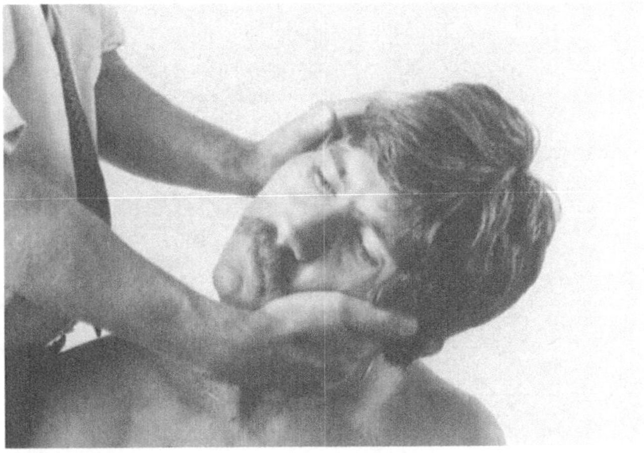

Fig. 64

Type of Treatment: Mobilization with impulse (thrust)
Goal: Improvement of sidebending at C2–C3
Technique: Rotation and sidebending manipulation
Therapeutic Usefulness: Great: FRG, AUS
Procedure: The cervical spine is flexed. Sidebending to one side is introduced (i.e. left). The patient's head rests against the operator's chest while the operator's right hand further fixes the hand by cradling the patient's chin. The operator's second metacarpal joint of the left hand is placed over the patient's left articular pillar of C2 (Fig. 65).
The impulse is effected through the left hand and is directed to the right and somewhat anteriorly.

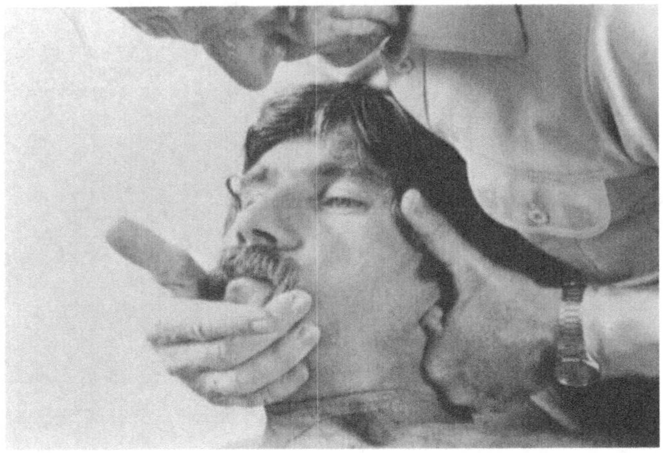

Fig. 65

Type of Treatment: Mobilization with impulse
Goal: Improvement of rotation at C2–C3
Technique: Rotation manipulation
Therapeutic Usefulness: Great: SWI
Procedure: The patient is sitting. The patient's head rests against the operator's thorax and is further stabilized with the operator's right hand. Maximum right rotation is introduced to the cervical spine. The operator places his metacarpal joint of the left index finger over the left articular pillar of C2 (Fig. 66).
The impulse follows right rotation and is effected through the second metacarpal joint on the left articular pillar of C2.

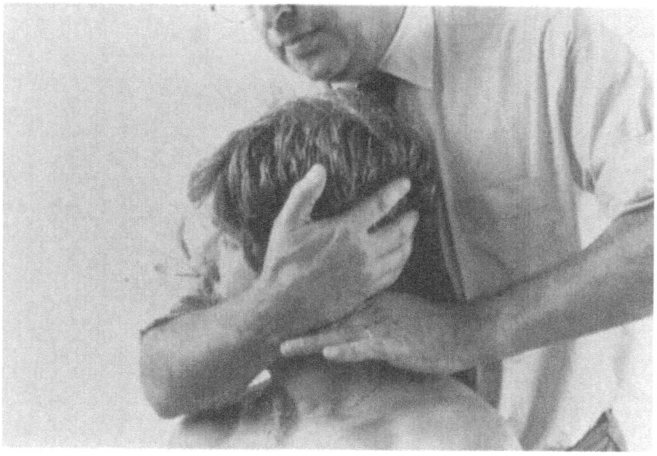

Fig. 66

Type of Treatment: Mobilization with impulse
Goal: Improvement of rotation at C2–C3
Technique: Rotation manipulation
Therapeutic Usefulness: Great: FRG
Procedure: The patient is supine and the cervical spine is flexed and sidebent to one side (i.e., left). The patient's head is stabilized by the operator cradling the chin and having the head rest against his thorax (Fig. 67).
The impulse, directed antero-laterally, is applied through the right proximal phalanx of the index finger.

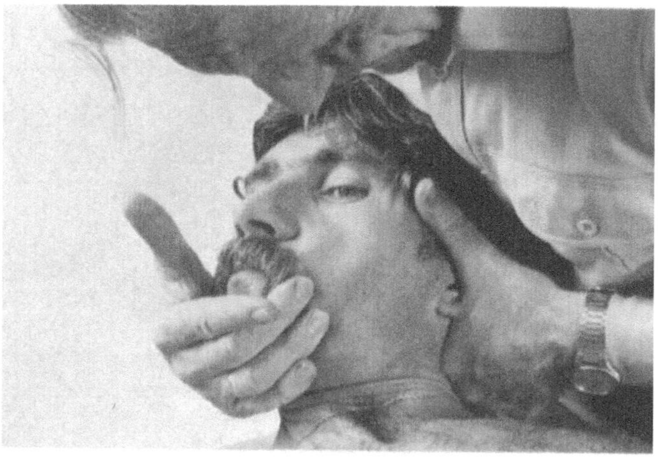

Fig. 67

Type of Treatment: Mobilization with impulse
Goal: Improvement of rotation at C2–C3
Technique: Rotation manipulation
Therapeutic Usefulness: Great: FRG, SWI
Procedure: The patient is sitting and the cervical spine is flexed. The articular pillar of C3 (i.e., left) is fixed with the operator's right thumb. The operator's fourth and fifth fingers are placed over the patient's right articular pillar of C2 (Fig. 68, 69).
The impulse is in direction of left rotation.

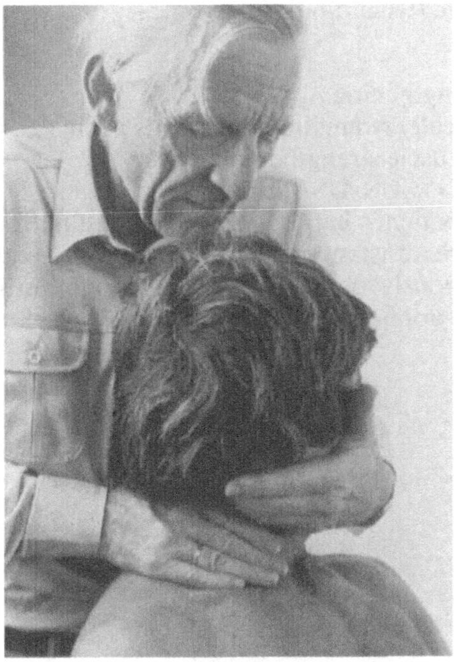

Fig. 68

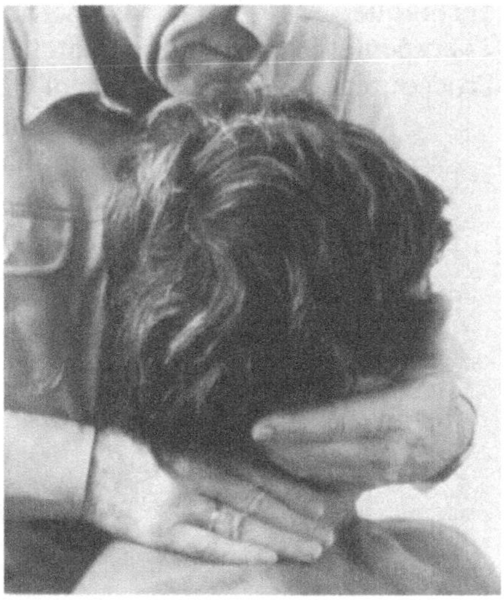

Fig. 69

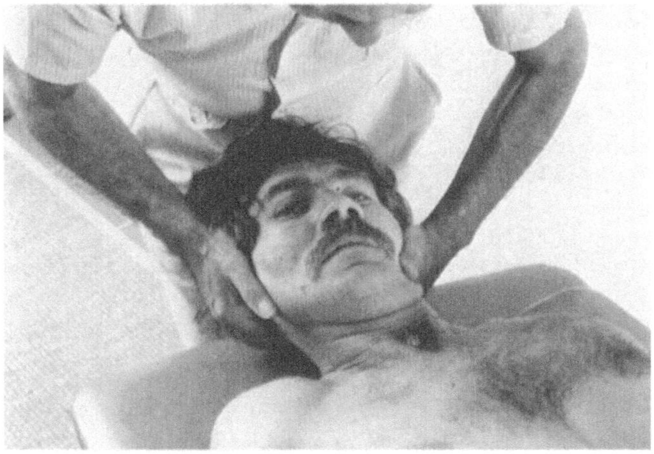

Fig. 70

Type of Treatment: Mobilization with impulse
Goal: Improvement of rotation at C1–C2 and C2–C3
Technique: Rotation manipulation
Therapeutic Usefulness: Great: AUS
Procedure: The patient is supine, and the cervical spine is flexed as well as rotated to one side (i.e., left). The proximal phalanx of the operator's index finger is placed over the articular pillar of C2 (Fig. 70). The impulse is along left rotation with some component directed superiorly.

3.4.4 Muscle Rehabilitation

Type of Treatment: Muscle strengthening
Goal: To isometrically strengthen the longus capitis and longus colli muscles
Technique: Isometric muscle strengthening
Therapeutic Usefulness: Great: FRG, AUS, USA, SWI
Procedure: One of the patient's hands is placed against his forehead so as to evoke minimal isometric resistance (the forehead pushes anteriorly). The cervical spine is simultaneously flexed (Fig. 71). This motion is monitored by the other hand which applies slight pressure in the anterior neck region.

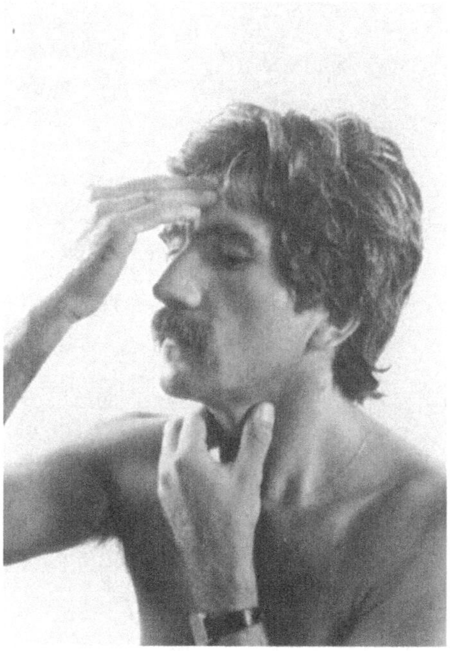

Fig. 71

Type of Treatment: Muscle stretching utilizing post-isometric relaxation.
Goal: Stretching of the suboccipital muscles.
Technique: Muscle stretch technique
Therapeutic Usefulness: Great: SWI, F, UK
Procedure: The articular pillars of C3 are fixed by one of the operator's hands in a vise-like manner. The head rests against the operator's thorax while the operator's free hand is placed over the patient's occiput (Fig. 72).
Passive flexion to the barrier is followed by isometric extension. During the relaxation phase there is mobilization by increasing the flexion component.

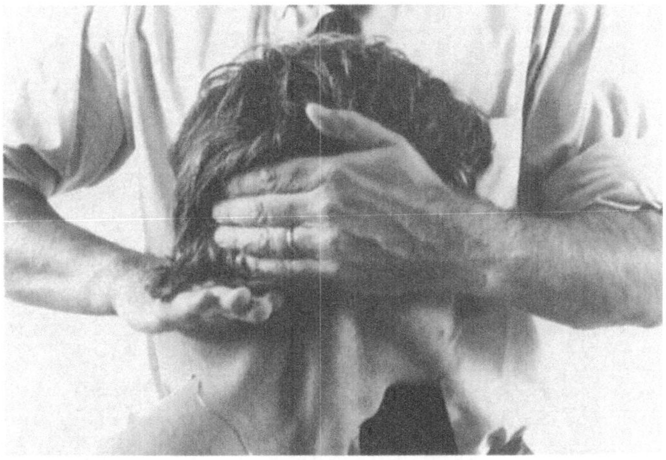

Fig. 72

Type of Treatment: Muscle stretching utilizing post-isometric relaxation.
Goal: Stretching of the suboccipital muscles.
Technique: Muscle stretch technique
Therapeutic Usefulness: Great: AUS
Moderate:
Little: USA, FRG
Procedure: With the patient supine maximum inclination is introduced, and the patient is fixed in this position. This is followed by isometric contraction of the extensor muscles. During the post-isometric relaxation phase passive stretching of the suboccipital muscle is accomplished by further flexing this section of the spine (Fig. 73).

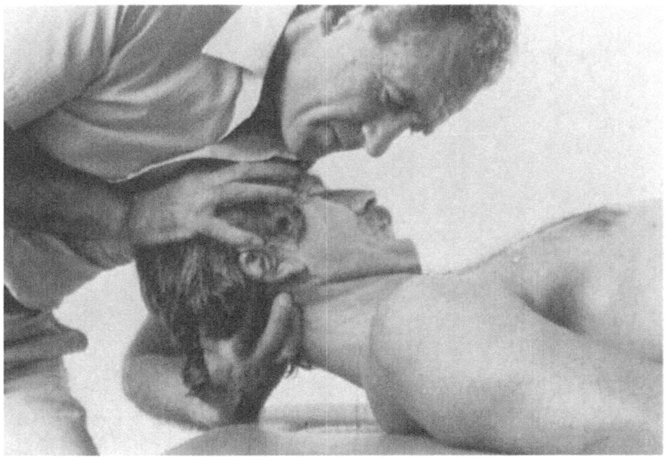

Fig. 73

Type of Treatment:	Muscle strengthening
Goal:	Strengthening of the anterior and posterior rectus muscles and the oblique muscles by isometric activation
Technique:	Muscle strengthening
Therapeutic Usefulness:	Great: FRG, AUS Moderate: USA, SWI None: F, UK
Procedure:	By either flexing or extending the segments C0–C1/C1–C2, isometric contraction is effected. The operator's hands provide the isometric counterforce specifically guiding the direction of the force (Figs. 74, 75).

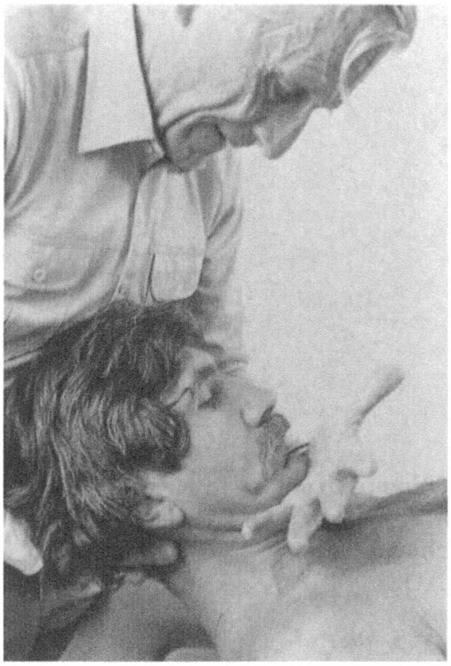

Fig. 74

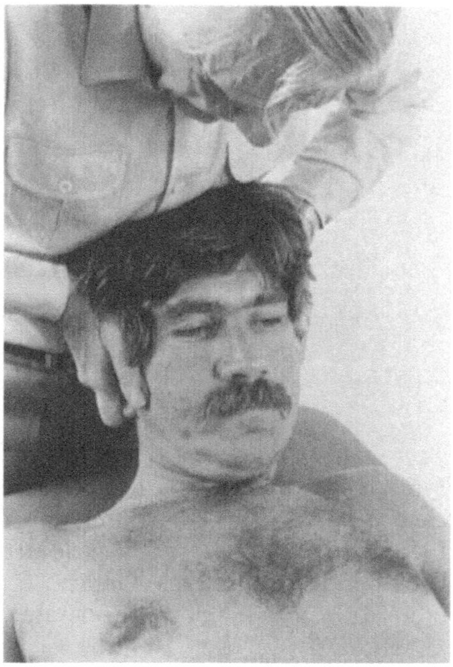

Fig. 75

Type of Treatment:	Muscle stretching utilzing post-isometric relaxation
Goal:	Stretching of the levator scapulae muscle
Technique:	Muscle stretch technique
Therapeutic Usefulness:	Great: FRG, AUS, USA, SWI
Procedure:	The scapulo-humeral joint is brought to its barrier through maximum elevation and internal rotation. The cervical spine is sidebent and rotated to one side. The operator's hand is placed flat over the cervical spine stabilizing it entirely. The patient is then instructed to contract the shoulder and arm muscles isometrically in a superior direction. The operator provides the resistant counterforce with his body. During the post-isometrical relaxation the levator scapulae muscle is stretched by the operator exerting pressure on the upper arm in the infero-posterior direction.

Type of Treatment:	Muscle stretching utilizing post-isometric relaxation
Goal:	Stretching of the trapezius muscle
Technique:	Muscle stretch technique
Therapeutic usefulness:	Great: FRG, AUS, USA, SWI

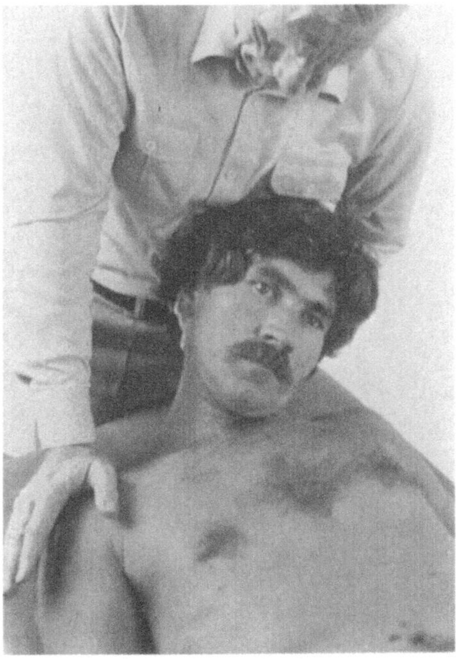

Fig. 76

Chapter 4

Mid-Cervical Spine, Cervico-Thoracic Junction and Ribs

Participants:

Austria (A): M. Berger
Czechoslovakia (CZE): V. Janda
Denmark (DEN): J. Foss-green
Switzerland (SWI): H. Trost
United Kingdom (UK): J. Patterson
USA: T. Allen, P. Kimberley
West Germany (FRG): A. Möhrle

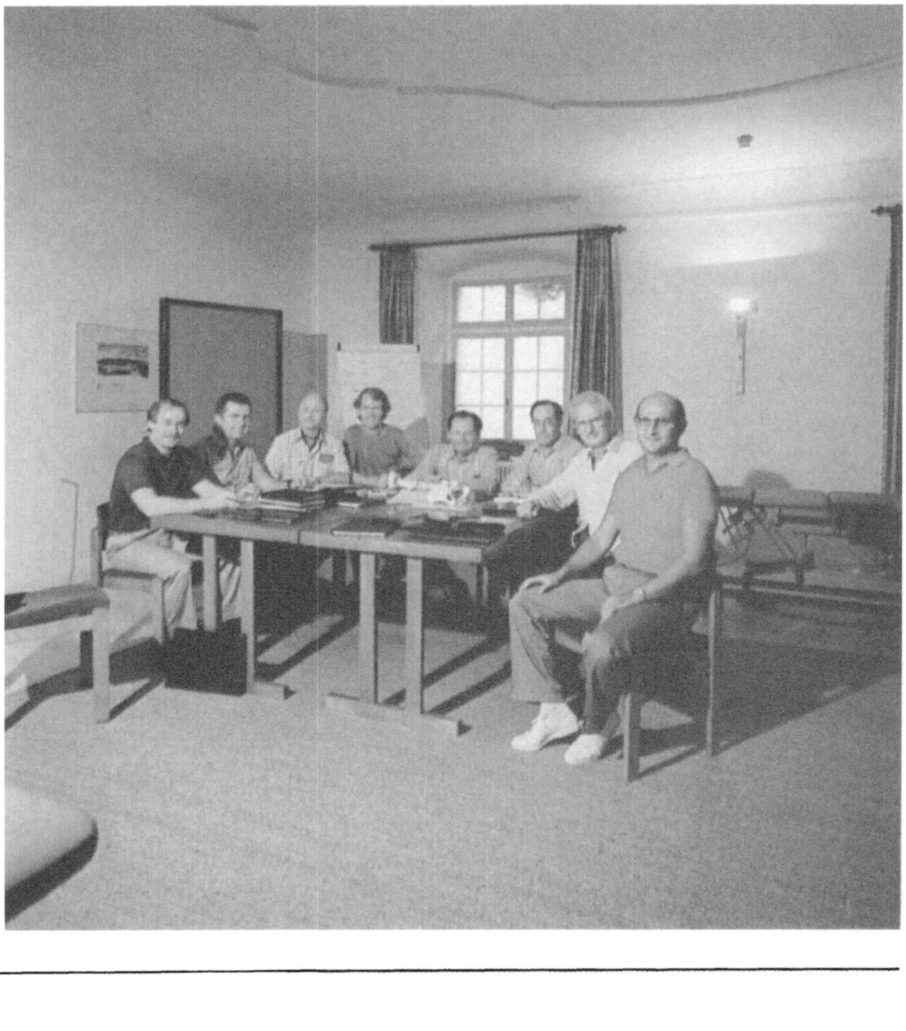

4.1 Mid-Cervical Spine and Cervico-Thoracic Junction – Biomechanical Considerations

The group agreed to include in their considerations of this spinal area (the cervico-thoracic junction) the vertebrae between C4 and T4, including ribs 1 to 4 and the thoracic inlet.
In order to better understand the function of this spinal area one should have a good anatomical and biomechanical knowledge. With the biomechanical aspects in mind, the more significant bony structures and their functional importance are considered herein.

4.1.1 Apophyseal Joints

The orientation of the facets of these joints changes from the mid-cervical spine to the upper thoracic spine, thus paralleling the functional changes in this region. In the lower cervical spine, the inclination of the facet plane is 45° to the horizontal plane, with the lower units showing a rather steep inclination as compared to the upper units (Fig. 77). The motions possible in each individual segment can be considered as the function of the combined translatory motions about each individual axis in the three-dimensional coordinate system. Rotation about the X-axis is identical to flexion-extension motions, rotation about the Y-axis in identical with axial rotation, and motion about the Z-axis coincides with sidebending (Fig. 78). Orientation of the thoracic apophyseal joint facets demonstrates inclination in two planes: starting with the horizontal plane, there is a rotation of 60° about the X-axis and 20° rotation about the Y-axis (Fig. 79). This arrangement of the two-fold inclination still allows rotation to take place in all three planes (flexion-extension, sidebending, and axial rotation). Sidebending in the cervical and thoracic spine are coupled with axial rotation (coupling patterns).

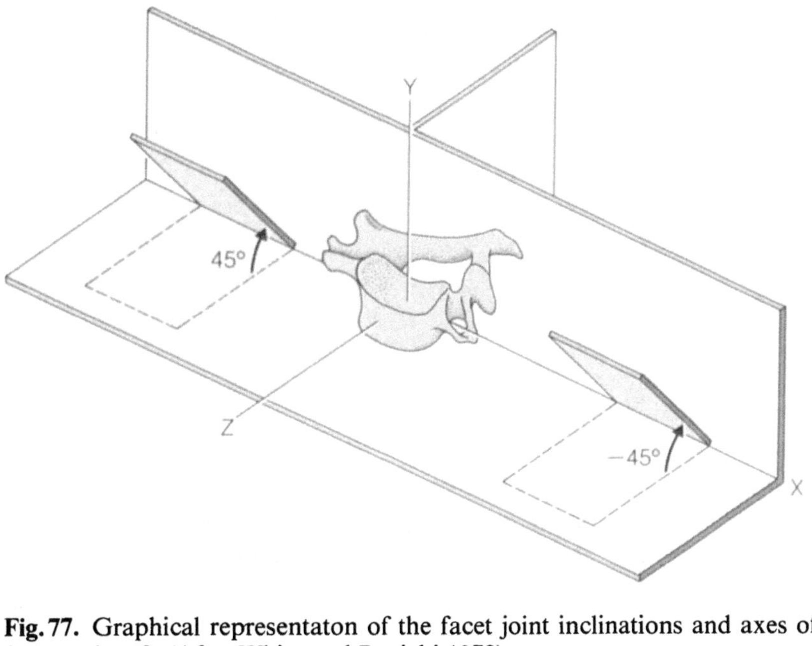

Fig. 77. Graphical representaton of the facet joint inclinations and axes of motion for vertebra C. (After White and Panjabi 1978)

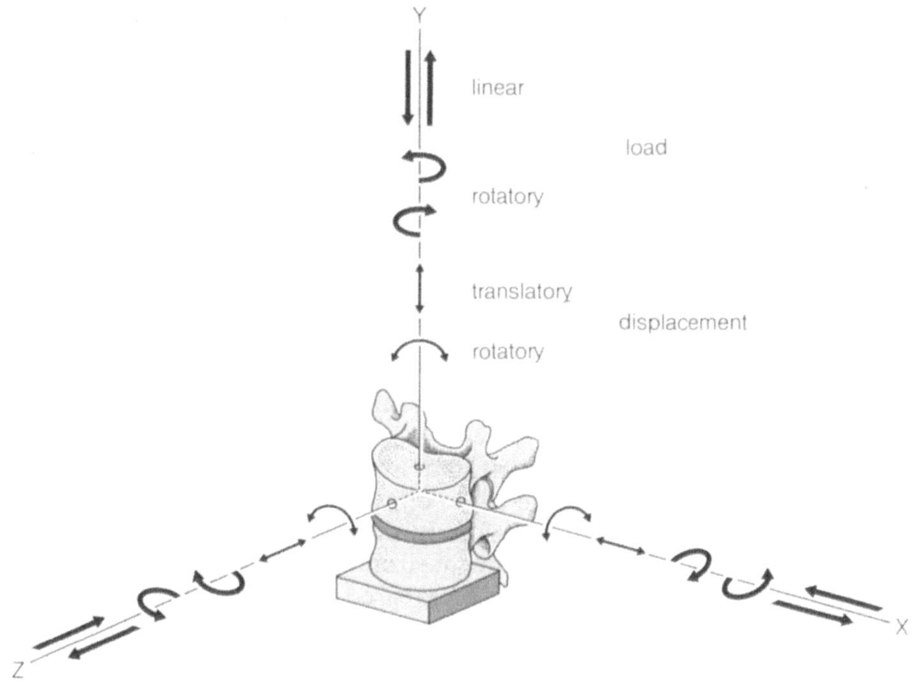

Fig. 78. A three-dimensional coordinate system has been placed at the center of the upper vertebral body of a vertebral unit (motion segment). A total of 12 load components, linear and rotatory, can act on these axes; the application of any one of the load components (linear or rotatory) produces displacement of the upper vertebra with respect to the lower vertebra. The displacement consists of translation and rotation (after White and Panjabi 1978)

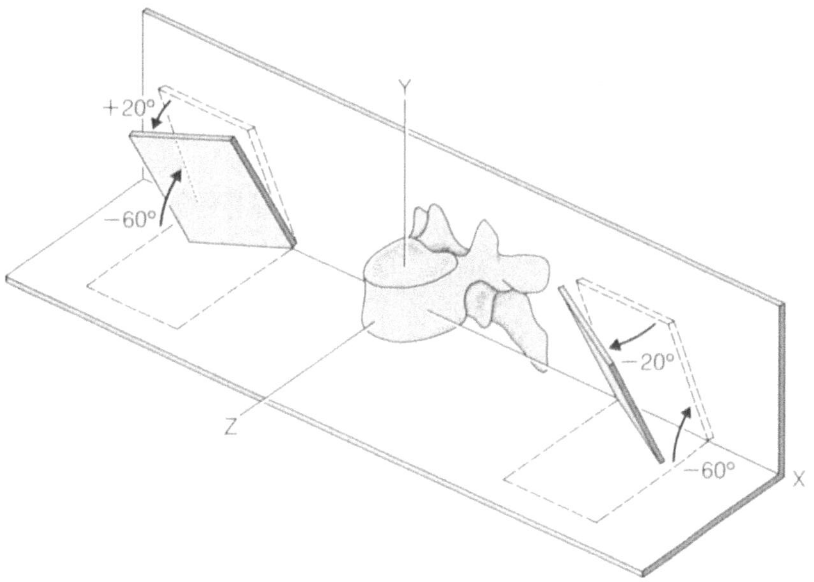

Fig. 79. Graphical representation of the facet joint inclinations and axes of motion of a thoracic vertebra (after White and Panjabi 1978)

4.1.2 Uncovertebral Joints

Even though one final opinion could not be reached as to these joints, a considerable amount of time was devoted to discussing their importance. These joints are not consistently developed. Some of the group's participants emphasized the protective action of the uncinate processes in regard to the intervertebral disk. One assumes that the fibrous joint capsule surrounding the uncovertebral joints display innervation similar to that of the apophyseal joints.
Degenerative changes are often seen in the uncinate processes and the uncovertebral joints which can possibly lead to chronic irritation of the nociceptive afferent fibers.

4.1.3 Soft Tissues

The Czechoslovakian school emphasized the importance of the functional pathology of the musculature affecting the harmonic motion patterns in all segments of the skeletal system. In the evaluation of muscular balance and especially imbalance, the physiological and functional aspects can be divided into two main groups, the phasic muscles and the postural muscles.
There was unanimity in that the problem of restricted motion should be approached both from a biomechanical standpoint – that is the structural changes of bones, joint capsules, and ligamentous apparatus as well as from a muscle-function standpoint considering the two important muscle groups. There exist indications that muscular balance disturbances have a more prominent impact on mobility than structural changes occurring in the bones themselves.
In contrast to the degenerative changes affecting the bony structures, muscular imbalance can be evaluated better and more importantly, it can be treated more successfully once the problem has been properly identified (including the patient's own exercises – self treatment).

4.2 Diagnosis

4.2.1 Diagnostic Criteria in the Assessment of Motion and Soft Tissues Relating to the Lower Cervical Spine and the Cervico-Thoracic Junction

After gross motion testing the cause of the segmental dysfunction affecting the cervico-thoracic junction is investigated. The evaluation specific to this segment consists of the following steps:

1. Gross Motion Testing

a) Inspected are
   - symmetry of the cervical spine,
   - symmetry of the upper and mid-thoracic spine,
   - symmetry of the thoracic inlet,

- shoulder levels,
- respiratory excursions,
- distance between the anterior and posterior axillary folds.

b) Regional gross motion testing
Active range of motion
Passive range of motion
- Quality of motion
- End feel of motion (gradual or abrupt barrier approach).

2. Soft Tissue and Skin Evaluation

a) Inspection
- skin color
- contours
- palpation – skin moisture
- palpatory evaluation of all connective tissue layers (skin, subcutaneous tissue, joint structures, and muscles). Distinctions are made as to quality differences (increased consistency, decreased plasticity, turgor, etc.).

b) Reaction to provocative testing
- subjective evaluation, pain induced upon palpation
- trigger points (zones of irritation)
- objective (vegetative stigmata).

3. Segmental Motion

- This includes in passive segmental examination evaluating mobility in 3 planes (X-axis: flexion-extension, Y-axis: axial rotation, Z-axis: sidebending).
- Evaluation of the intervertebral joints (joint play, translatory movement).
- Joints involving the ribs
- Joints of the shoulder girdle, including the acromio-clavicular the sterno-clavicular joints.

4. Muscle Function Testing

The tests for muscle function should be carried out in a systematic approach concentrating on regional muscle groups.
The following muscles should be assessed routinely: trapezius muscle (descending and horizontal portions), levator scapulae muscle, semispinalis capitis muscle, rhomboid major and minor muscles, deltoid muscle, anterior serratus muscle, sternocleidomastoid muscle, scalene muscles, longus colli and longus capitis muscles.
Frequently one finds increased tone, functional muscle shortening or painful mytendinoses (trapezius muscle, levator scapulae muscle, pectoralis major and minor muscles, sternocleidomastoid muscle). These muscles belong phylogenetically to the old postural muscles.
In the primarily phylogenetically young muscles which participate mainly in phasic functions, one finds diminished strength. This can be typically seen in

the deltoid muscle, rhomboid muscles, serratus anterior muscle, and especially the horizontal portion of the trapezius muscle.
Muscular imbalance (shortening of the postural muscles and weakening of the phasic muscles), which is a frequent finding, can lead to rotation and elevation of the shoulder blades as well as to an increased distance between the inferior angle of the scapula and the spinous processes.

5. Functional Examination of Respiratory Excursion

In addition to the inspection of the respiratory excursion, one uses palpation to evaluate the movement of the individual ribs during inspiration and expiration so as to determine if any dysfunction are present.

4.2.2 Soft Tissue Examination

Spinal Area: Cervico-thoracic junction
Type of Examination: Palpatory examination of skin and subcutaneous tissues
Diagnostic Usefulness: Great: CZE, DEN, SWI, FRG, UK
Procedure: A fold of skin and subcutaneous tissue is formed between the operator's thumb and index finger and is moved over some area (Kibler-fold). Evaluated are changes in skin turgor and thus the fold's thickness as is the patient's pain perception (Fig. 80).

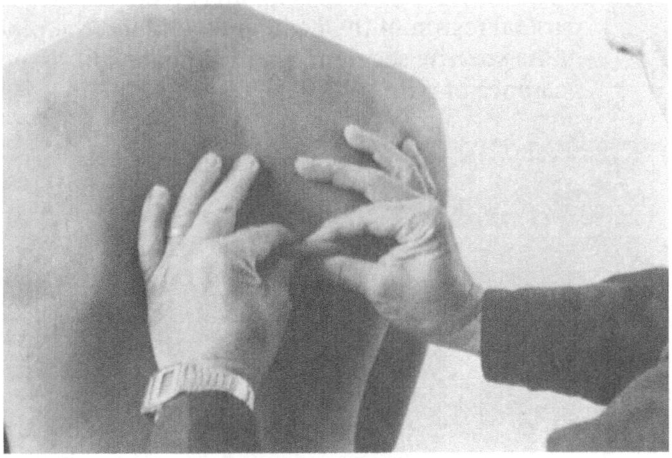

Fig. 80

Spintal Area: C2–T6
Type of Examination: Segmental zones of irritation
Diagnostic Usefulness: Great: SWI, DEN, USA
None: FRG

Procedure: Of practical importance is the zone of irritation located at the superior articular process. The 4 fingers of the palpating hand are first placed over the spinous processes of C2–C6 and, in a hook-like manner, reach around the strong semispinalis capitis muscle, then they encounter a groove which is formed by the semispinalis capitis and the longissimus capitis muscles. The palpating fingers should establish as close a bony contact as possible so that they can actually feel the superior articular process which can be perceived as a slight protuberance. In the neutral position, the superior articular process of C2 is one finger-width below the occiput and about one finger-width superior to the inferior edge of the spinous process of C2 (Fig. 81). When the neck is maximally extended, the zone of irritation of C4 is located at the lowest point of the concave cervical spine. Local tissue changes and painful pressure points are palpated for and evaluated.

The zone of irritation at C7 is more difficult to palpate mainly due to the strong fibers of the trapezius muscle and the long back muscles. The transverse and spinous process of C7 (vertebra prominens) are located first. The zone of irritation is found two finger-widths above the spinous process and about one finger-width medial to the tip of the transverse process (Fig. 82).

All zones of irritation in the cervical spine react upon provocative testing. A decrease of pain perception or any tissue change indicates the correct therapeutic direction for the segment in question. The palpating index or middle finger rests on the zone of irritation applying constant pressure. The pressure is such that the patient can barely feel the pain. The other hand embraces the parietal region of the head and conducts the physiological motions possible in the specific segment. Evaluated are soft tissue changes as well as the appearance of pain.

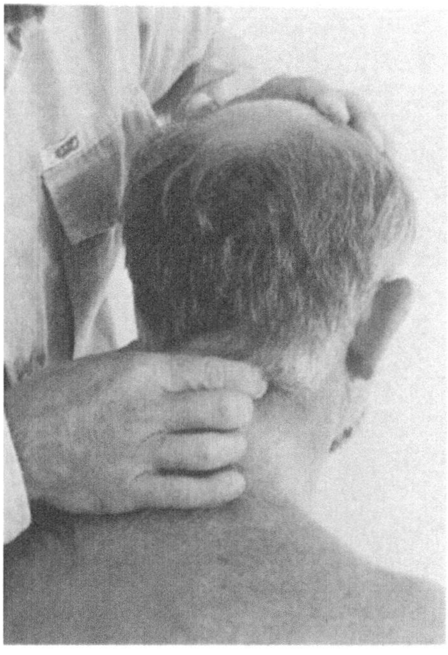
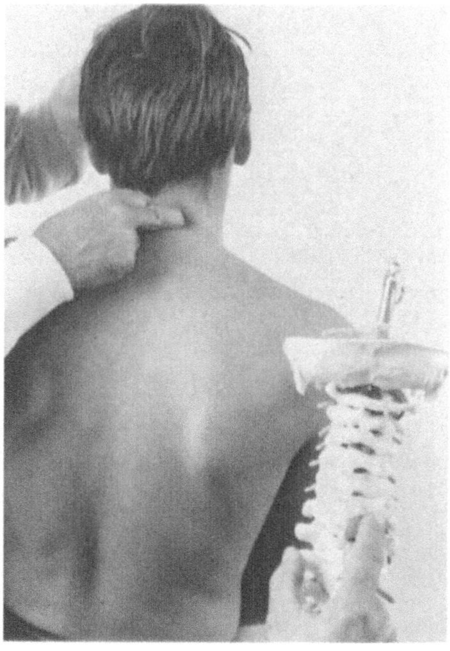

Fig. 81 **Fig. 82**

4.2.3 Motion Testing

Spinal Area: C6–C7 to T5–T6

Type of Examination: Segmental examination of flexion and extension motions in the cervical spine via the spinous processes.

Diagnostic Usefulness: Great: DEN, CZE, SWI, FRG

Procedure: The operator stands behind the upright sitting patient and flexes the patient's head with one hand. The finger of the palpating hand is placed segmentally over adjoining spinous processes. Passive flexion-extension motions of the neck are then introduced, and one evaluates the range of motion and compares the mobility of the individual processes against each other (Figs. 83, 84).

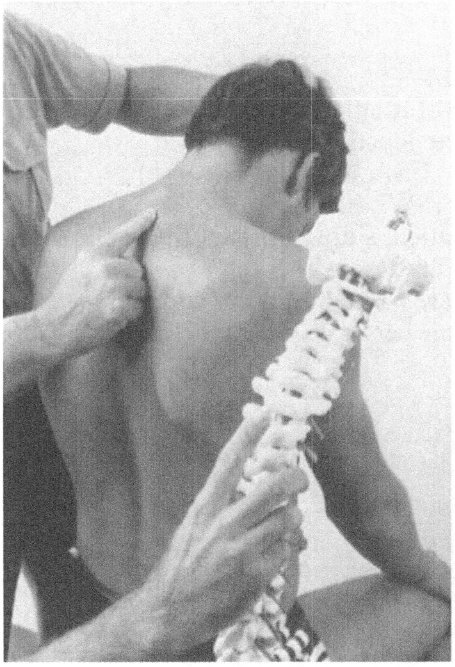

Fig. 83

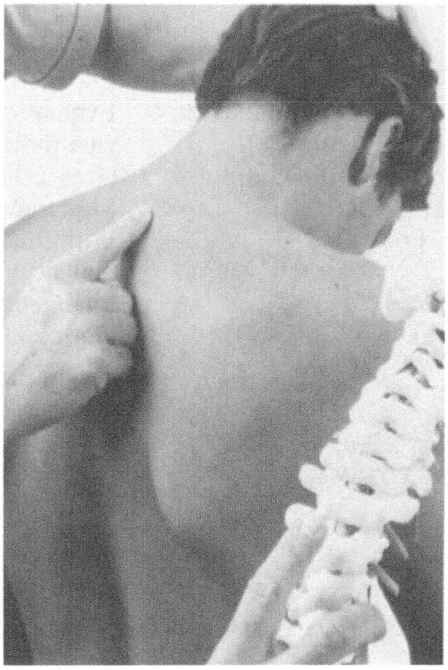

Fig. 84

Spinal Area: C6–C7 to T4–T5

Type of Examination: Segmental examination of side-bending motions.

Diagnostic Usefulness: Great: USA, CZE, FRG, DEN, SWI

Procedure: The patient is in the upright sitting position; while one hand of the operator introduces sidebending to the neck, the index and middle fingers of the other hand palpate the apophyseal joints on the concave side (Fig. 85). Evaluated are range of motion and end feel seen during the motion in the individual segments.

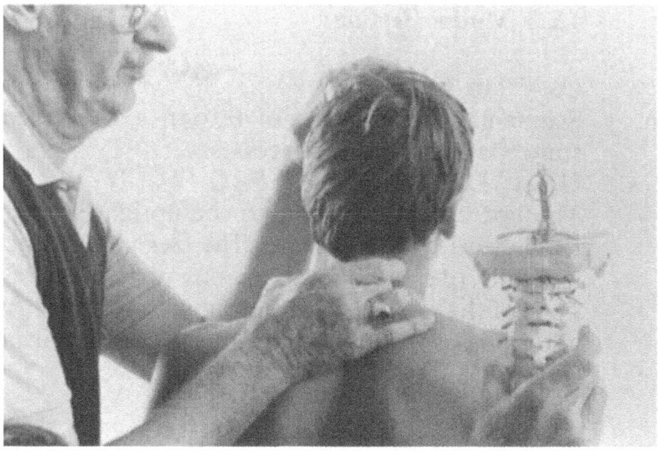

Fig. 85

Spinal Area: C4–C5 to T4–T5

Type of Examination: Evaluation of rotation motions in the entire cervical spine including the cervico-thoracic junction.

Diagnostic Usefulness: Great: USA, CZE, DEN
Moderate: SWI, FRG

Procedure: With the patient sitting upright, the cervical spine is rotated passively to either side (Fig. 86).
Evaluated are range of motion and end feel. The normal rotational range of motion of the cervical spine is 90° to either side.

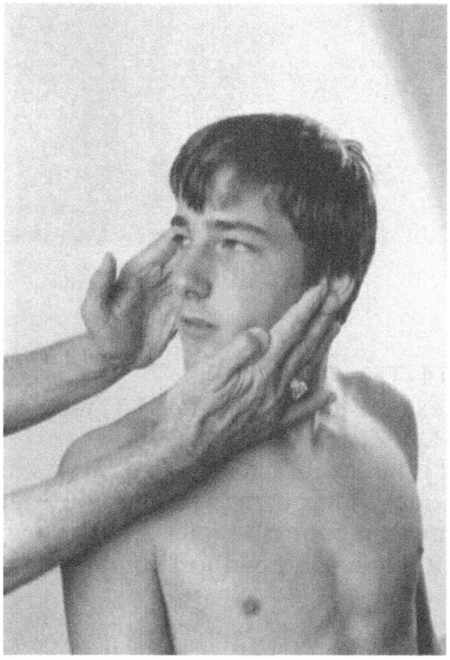

Fig. 86

Spinal Area: C4–C5 to T3–T4

Type of Examination: Gross motion testing of the lower cervical spine and the cervico-thoracic junction (rotation of the head while the cervical spine is extended).

Diagnostic Usefulness: Great: SWI, CZE
Moderate: FRG

Procedure: The patient is sitting upright. The patient's head is embraced in the parietal regions with both hands and is then passively extended (Fig. 87). The upper cervical joints (C0–C1–C2) are thus brought into a position whereby further motion is prevented. Passive rotation of the head coupled with slight side-bending is then only possible in the lower segments of the cervical spine. An empirical normal value for some such motion is given as 60° to either side.

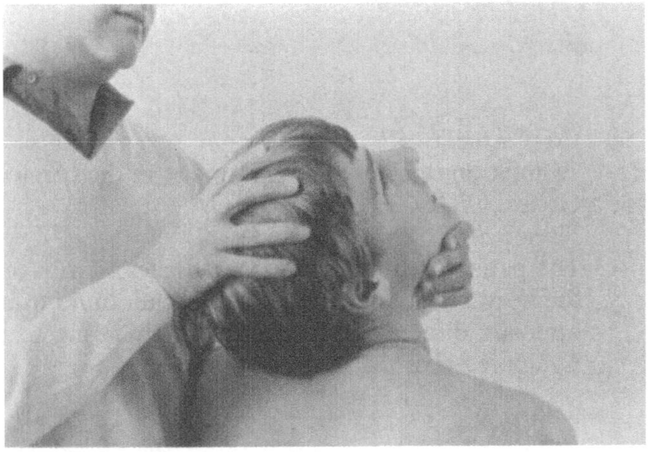

Fig. 87

Spinal Area: C6–C7 to T2–T3

Type of Examination: Segmental testing of rotation and sidebending motions.

Diagnostic Usefulness: Great: SWI, DEN

Procedure: The patient is sitting upright with the cervical spine held in the neutral position. The head is then slightly rotated and sidebent (Fig. 88). The palpating fingers are resting on the spinous processes evaluate the range of motion in the individual segments (Fig. 89).

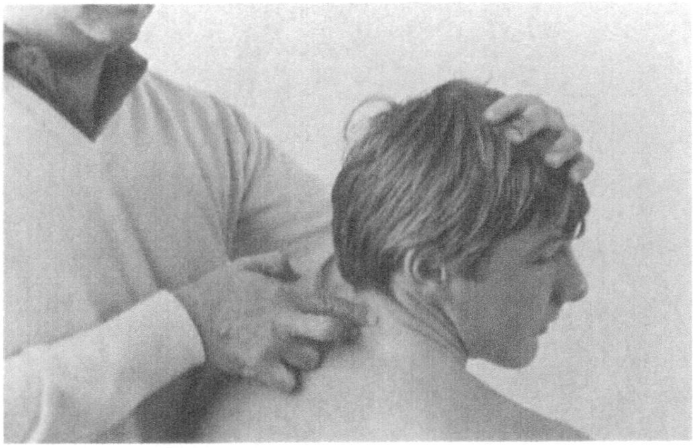

Fig. 88

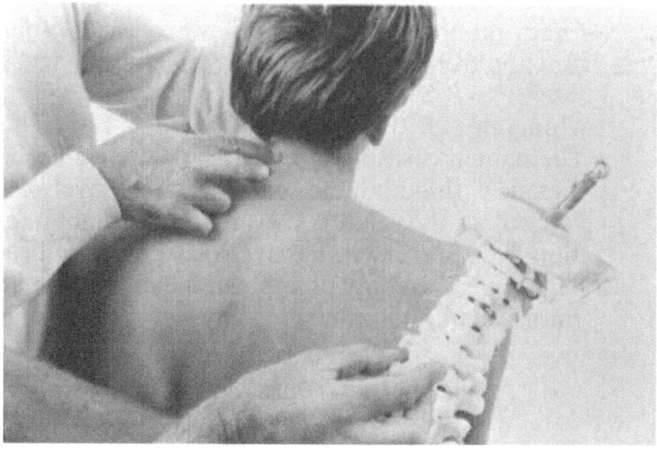

Fig. 89

Spinal Area: C6–C7 to T6–T7

Type of Examination: Evaluation of sidebending motions in the cervico-thoracic junction.

Diagnostic Usefulness: Great: USA, CZE, DEN, FRG

None: SWI

Procedure: The patient is sitting. The operator leans with one arm on the shoulder and the head of the patient while the other hand translates the shoulder into the opposite direction introducing sidebending to the cervical spine (Fig. 90). Evaluated is of the range of motion.

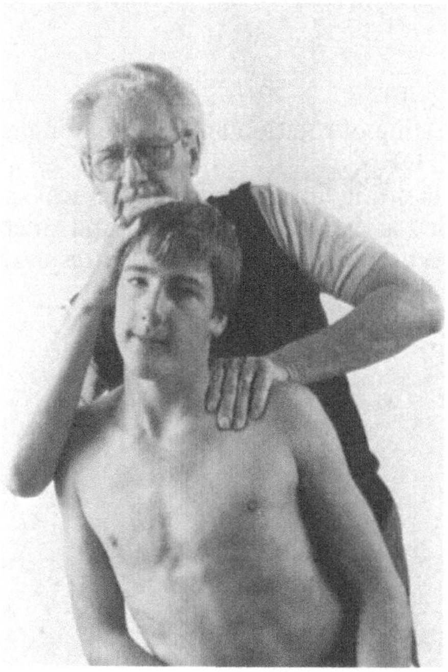

Fig. 90

Spinal Area: C4–C5 to C7/T1

Type of Examination: Segmental translatory examination of the lower cervical spine in flexion and extension.

Diagnostic Usefulness: Great: USA, FRG, CZE

Procedure: The patient is supine. The fingertips of the palpating fingers rest over the apophyseal joints. The operator introduces translatory motion to each individual segment. Evaluated are the ease of the translations, quality and end feel (Fig. 91). This procedure is carried out both with the neck flexed and extended (Fig. 92).

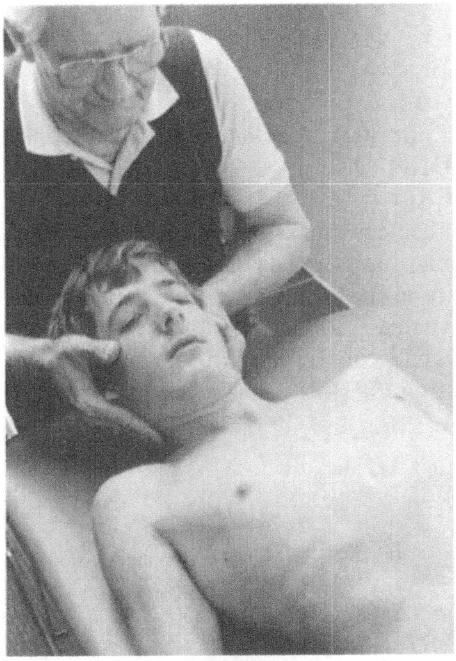

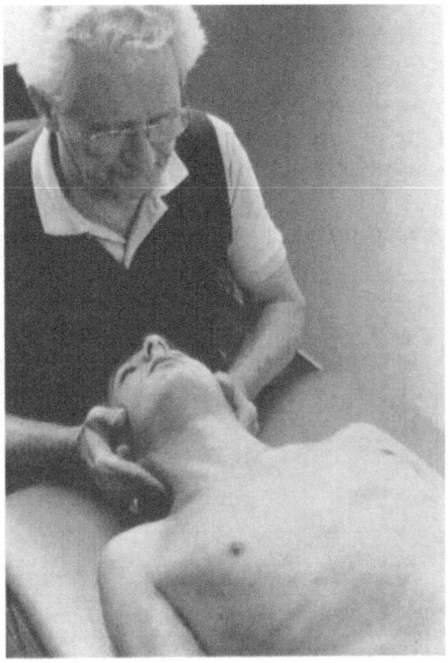

Fig. 91 Fig. 92

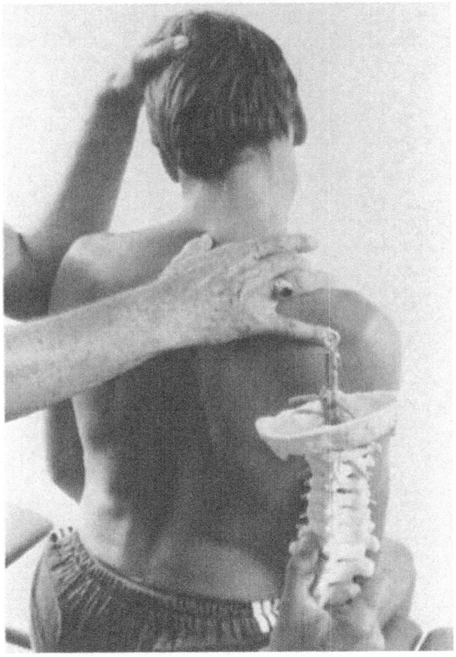

Fig. 93

Spinal Area: C4–C5 to T4–T5
Type of Examination: Evaluation of translatory and coupled motions in the cervical spine and the cervico-thoracic junction
Diagnosis Usefulness: Great: USA
Procedure: The patient is sitting. The operator places his right thumb and index finger over the apophyseal joints of a spinal segment while his left hand is placed on the patient's head and the left elbow comes to rest on the patient's shoulder (Fig. 93).
With the patient completely relaxed the operator's right hand introduces a translatory motion in the individual spinal segment. The ease of translatory motion is evaluated both in maximal flexion and extension.

Spinal Area: C3–C4 to C7–T1
Type of Examination: Evaluation of coupled motions in the lower cervical spine
Diagnosis Usefulness: Great: DEN
Moderate: FRG
Procedure: The operator places his index finger over the apophyseal joint and the thumb on the spinous process of the same spinal segment. With the ulnar border of his other hand the operator stabilizes the vertebra above in particular and with the rest of his hand the other vertebrae above as well (Figs. 94, 95). Combined flexion, sidebending and rotation to the same side is introduced evaluating the positional relationship of the articular surfaces to each other.

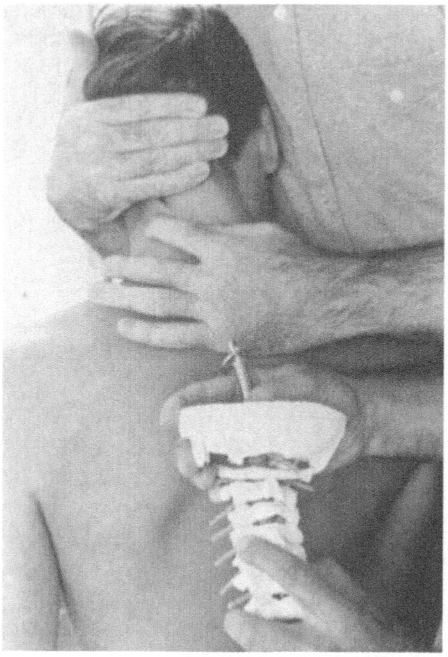
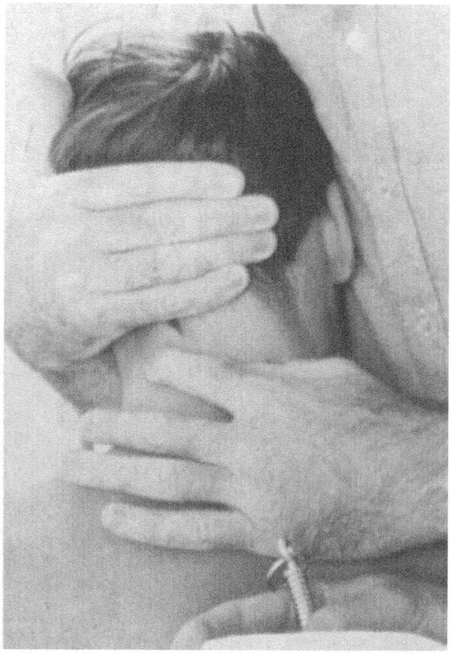

Fig. 94 **Fig. 95**

Spinal Area: T1–T2 to T4–T5

Type of Examination: Gross motion testing.

Diagnostic Usefulness: Great: USA, DEN, CZE
None: SWI

Procedure: The patient is sitting upright. The examiner places his/her hands on the patient's shoulder and then introduces maximal passive rotation of the upper body (Figs. 96, 97).
Evaluated are range of motion and quality of the barrier.

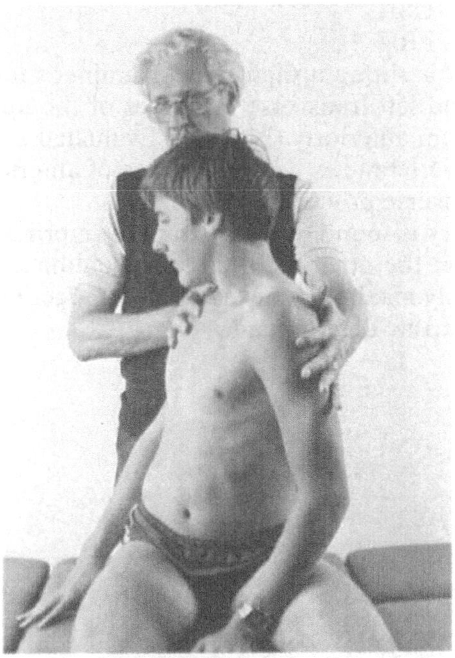
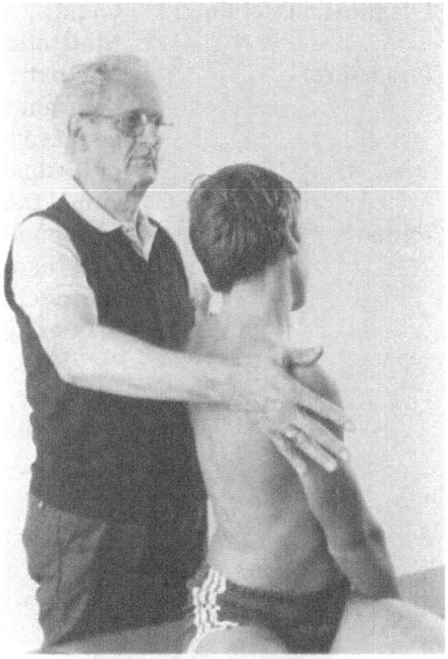

Fig. 96 Fig. 97

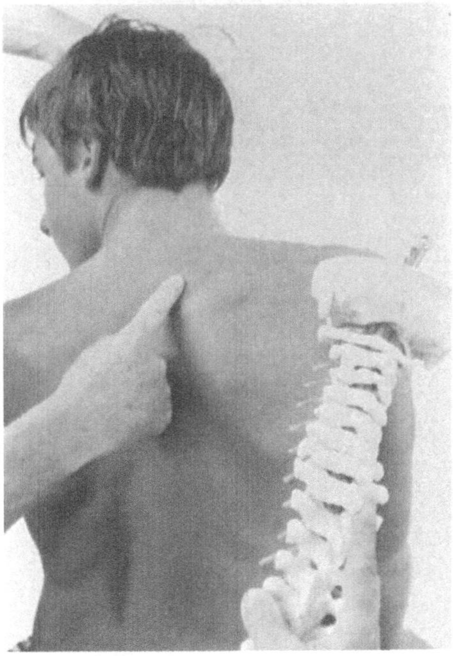
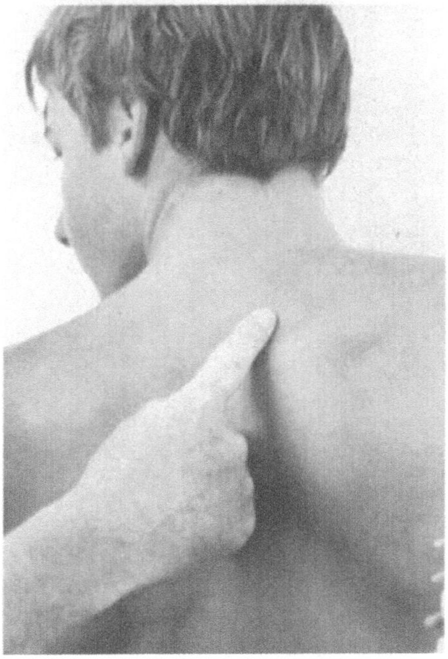

Fig. 98 Fig. 99

Spinal Area:	C7–T1 to T4–T5
Type of Examination:	Segmental rotation testing musing spinous process.
Diagnostic Usefulness:	Great: DEN, CZE, SWI, FRG, UK
Procedure:	The examiner stands behind the sitting patient. While one hand introduces passive maximal rotation of the head the palpating finger rests on the spinous processes (Figs. 98, 99), and evaluates motion of the spinous processes in relation to adjacent vertebral units.

Spinal Area:	T1–T2 to T4–T5
Type of Examination:	Segmental evaluation of rotation movement.
Diagnostic Usefulness:	Great: USA Moderate: FRG
Procedure:	The patient is sitting upright. The examiner's thumbs palpate alternatingly the right and left transverse processes of the upper thoracic vertebrae and displace them anteriorly (Fig. 100). Evaluated are positional changes of the individual vertebrae as well as the ease of anterior displacement of the individual transverse processes.
Remarks:	If asymmetry is found (i.e., one transverse process is more posterior on one side than on the other side) the examination is repeated with the cervical spine actively maximally flexed and extended. Presence of asymmetry is the major diagnositc determinant.

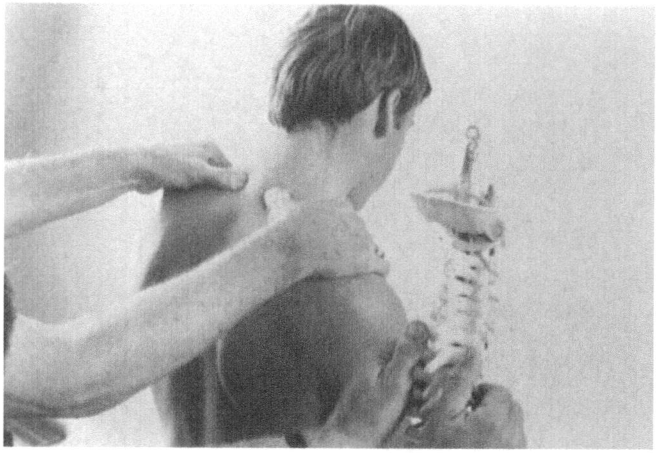

Fig. 100

Spinal Area: Acromio-clavicular joint
Type of Examination: Motion testing of this joint, passive gapping.
Diagnostic Usefulness: Moderate: USA
Procedure: The examiner stands behind the sitting patient. The index finger of the examining hand palpates the joint space of the acromio-clavicular joint. The elbow of the same side is brought anteriorly and medially in front of the thorax with simultaneous slight rotation in the shoulder joint while the arm is abducted (Fig. 101). This procedure causes the acromio-clavicular joint to gap. Evaluated are the range of motion and joint play.

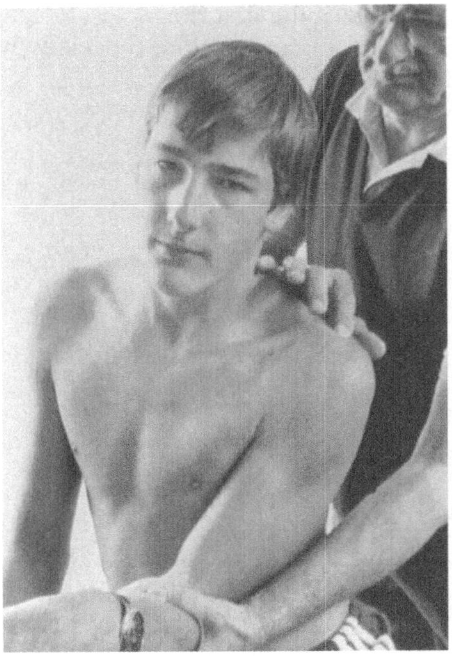

Fig. 101

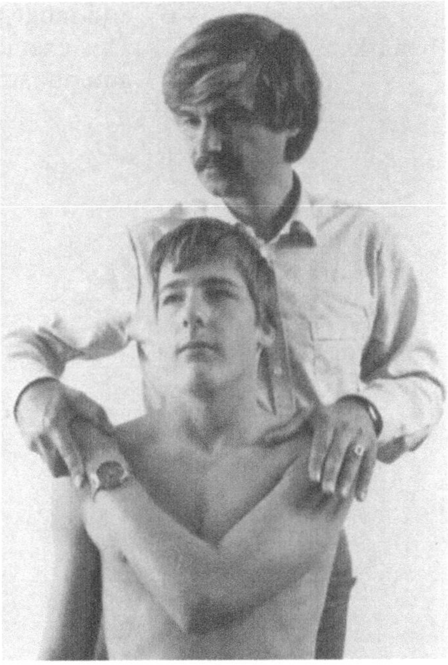

Fig. 102

Spinal Area: Acromio-clavicular Joint
Type of Examination: Motion testing of this joint.
Diagnostic Usefulness: Great: AUS
Moderate: CZE, SWI
Procedure: The examiner stands behind the sitting patient. While one hand of the examiner fixes the shoulder of the patient, the other hand guides the patient's arm passively over the opposite shoulder (Fig. 102). Evaluated are range of motion of the arm and joint play in the acromio-clavicular joint.

Spinal Area: First rib

Type of Examination: Motion testing of the first rib.

Diagnostic Usefulness: Great: AUS, CZE, SWI, FRG

Procedure: The examiner stands behind the upright sitting patient. The cervical spine is flexed passively, rotated to the opposite side and sidebent to the same side (modification for Switzerland and Germany: the cervical spine is passively rotated and sidebent to the same side). Pressing the descending portion of the trapezius muscle posteriorly, the palpating hand (index finger) is placed along the superior surface of the first rib so as to establish as large a contact area as possible (Fig. 103). With good bony contact a springing force is introduced in the direction of the opposite upper thigh. Evaluated are the ease and range of motion of the first rib.

Remarks: This examination often causes pain, especially when myotendinoses of the anterior scalene muscle are present.

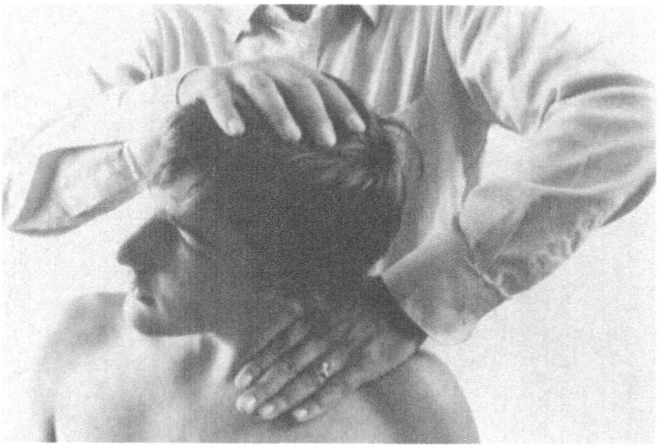

Fig. 103

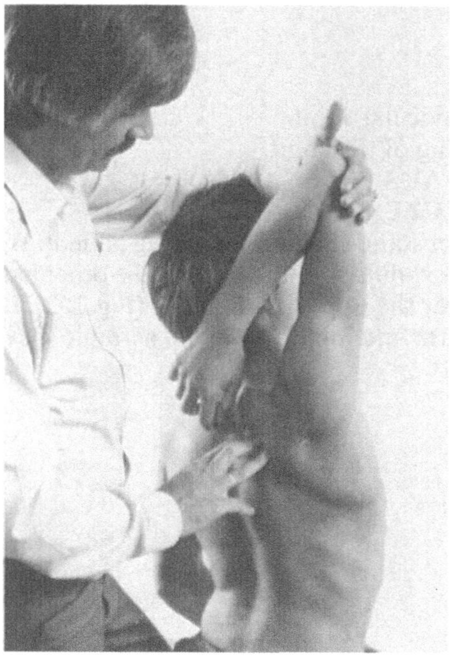

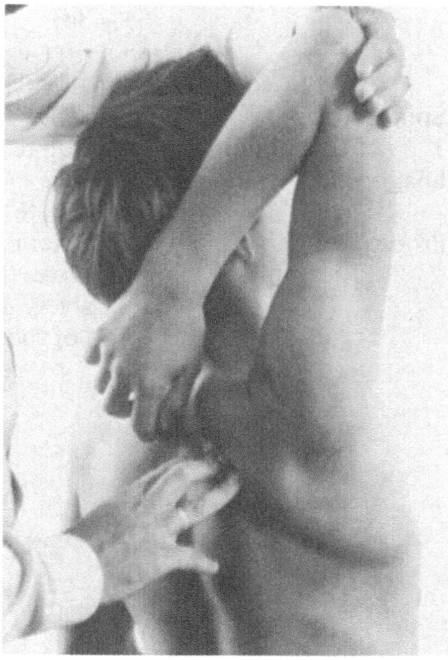

Fig. 104 **Fig. 105**

Spinal Area: Thoracic Inlet
Type of Examination: Motion testing for upper ribs.
Diagnostic Usefulness: Great: AUS
Moderate: CZE

Procedure: The operator stands behind and at the side of the upright sitting patient. The patient reaches with his hand for the neck region while elevating, externally rotating and abducting the arm in the shoulder joint. In a similar fashion, the patient's elbow is guided superiorly while the fingers of the operator palpate the vertebral portions of the upper ribs (Fig. 104, 105). The patient is requested to deeply inhale and exhale. Evaluated are motion of the individual ribs.

4.2.4 Neuromuscular Examination

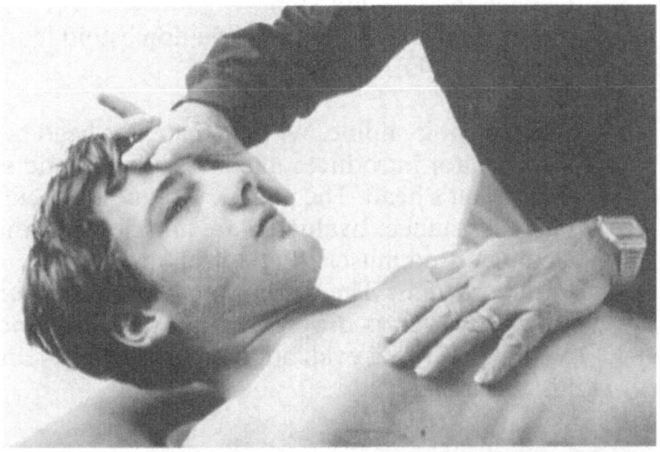

Fig. 106

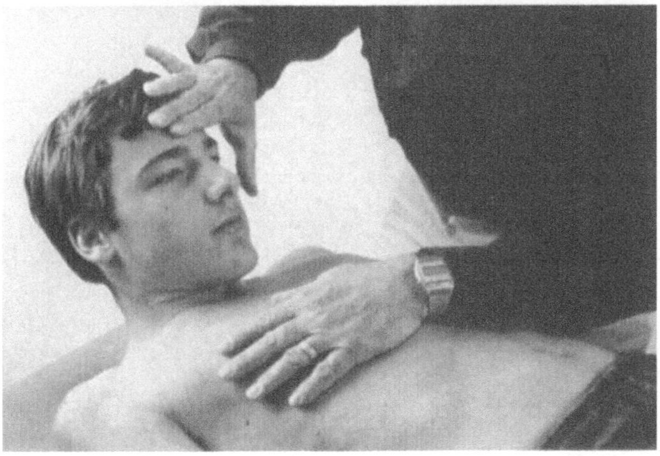

Fig. 107

Spinal Area: C4–T4

Type of Examination: Examination of the deep cervical spine flexor muscles (longus colli muscle, longus capitis muscle)

Diagnostic Usefulness: Great: CZE, SWI, DEN
Moderate: FRG

Procedure: The patient is supine. While the examiner stabilizes with his right hand the patient's thorax, the left hand exerts a slight counterforce on the forehead (Fig. 106). The patient is requested to flex his head. One analyses and evaluates primarily the beginning of this motion (Fig. 107).

Pathological Findings: If the deep neck flexor muscles are weakened, the patient is unable to lift his head and pushes the chin anteriorly by activating the sternocleidomastoid muscle instead. Weakening would also lead to a reclination motion in the occiput-atlas articulation.

Spinal Area: Cervico-thoracic junction

Procedure: Strength testing of the sternocleidomastoid muscle.

Diagnosis Usefulness: Great: DEN, SWI
Moderate: CZE

Procedure: The patient is supine. With the patient's head beyond the examination table, the operator introduces maximal rotation and simultaneous sidebending to the patient's head. The patient is requested to lift his head against the examiner's resistance. Evaluated are muscle strength and contours of the sternocleidomastoid muscle (Fig. 108).
Variation CZE: The starting position is the same as described above; the head, however, is dropped under guidance and brought into further sidebending allowing evaluation of stretchability and painfulness of the muscle insertions.

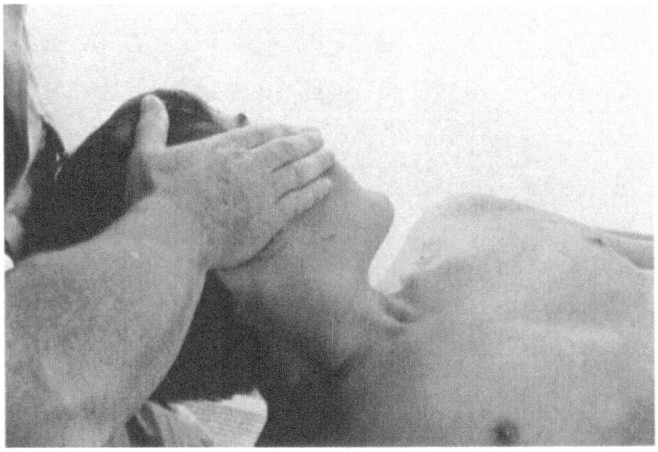

Fig. 108

Spinal Area: Cervico-thoracic junction
Procedure: Palpation of the trapezius muscle.
Diagnosis Usefulness: Great: SWI, FRG, CZE, DEN
Procedure: Due to its subcutaneous position, the trapezius muscle, in particular its descending portion, is easily accessible for palpation and should provide little difficulty for even the beginner. The anatomical arrangement of all of its components is well defined. First, the thumb and index finger take hold of the muscle belly (the descending portion of the muscle) halfway between shoulder and neck and then palpate perpendicularly to its fibers' orientation (Fig. 109). In the second step, the muscle insertions are palpated. Following the muscle's fibers direction carefully, the tendinoses can be palpated over the spinous processes, the spine of the scapula and the clavicle (Fig. 110).
Remarks: The trapezius muscle is of special importance in the routine diagnosis of the spondylogenic reflex syndrome. Not uncommonly can functional disturbances (somatic dysfunctions) encountered in the thoracic spine cause individual muscle bundles to undergo painful pathological changes (myotendinoses).

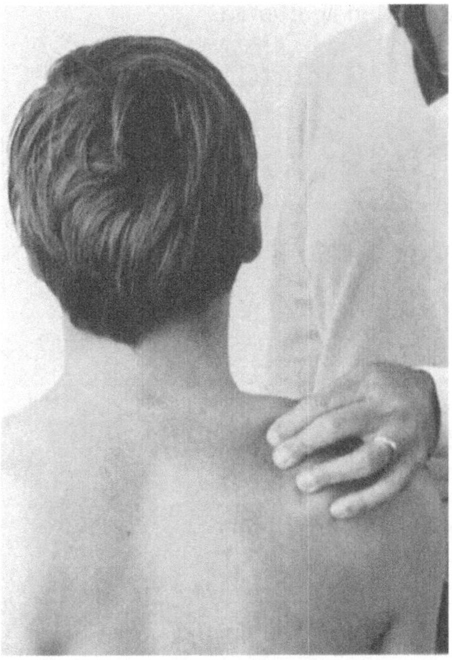

Fig. 109

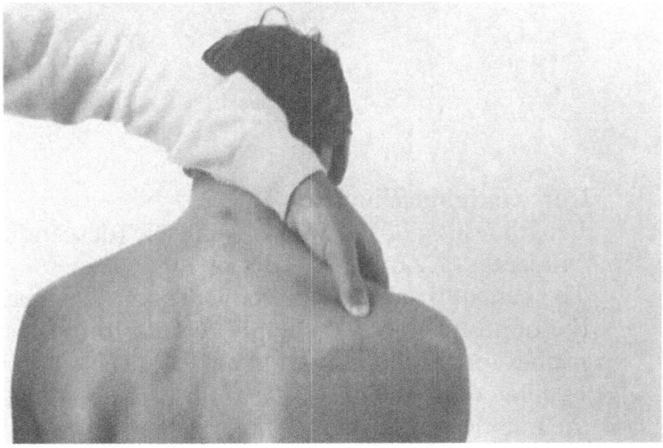

Fig. 110

Spinal Area: Cervico-thoracic junction
Type of Examination: Length testing of the levator scapulae muscle
Diagnostic Usefulness: Great: CZE, SWI, FRG
Moderate: DEN
Procedure: The patient is supine. The operator cradles the patient's neck with one hand and rests the head on his forearm. The cervical spine is passively flexed, rotated to one side and sidebent to the opposite side. The head stays fixed in this position throughout the examination.
The operator introduces a rotation of the scapula about a sagittal axis. This can be done in the following way: the examiner either moves the shoulder with the scapula inferiorly or he passively elevates and externally rotates the patient's arm so as to place it under the patient's head (Fig. 111).
Evaluated are the elasticity and length of the levator scapulae muscle.
With his thumb, the operator simultaneously follows the muscle fibers to the point of the levator scapulae muscle's insertion (medial superior edge of the scapula) (Fig. 112). One evaluates whether painful insertion tendinoses are present; when palpating perpendicularly to the muscle fibers' direction at the level of C7 for instance, one may encounter painful myoses.
Remarks: The muscle is often shortened.

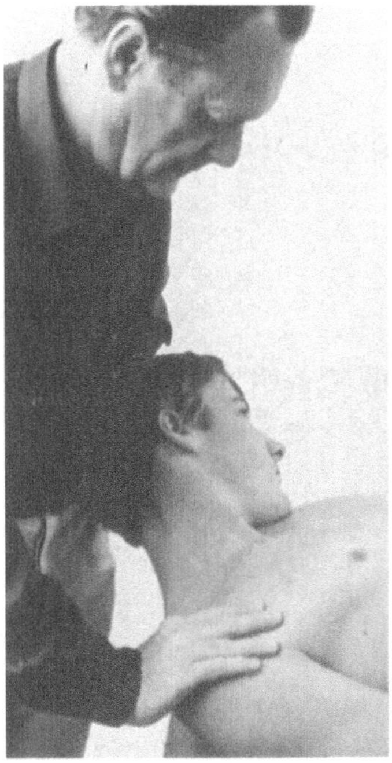
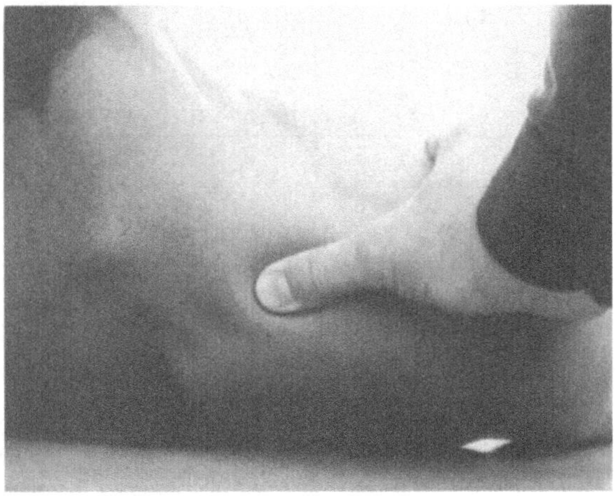

Fig. 111 **Fig. 112**

Spinal Area: Cervico-thoracic junction
Type of Examination: Length testing of the trapezius muscle (descending portion):
Diagnostic Usefulness: Moderate: CZE, SWI, DEN
Procedure: The patient is supine. The cervical spine is flexed and the head is sidebent to the opposite side and slightly rotated to the ipsilateral side. The examiner pushes the shoulder inferiorly (Fig. 113).
Evaluated are the elasticity of the trapezius muscle as well as symmetry of the muscle contours.

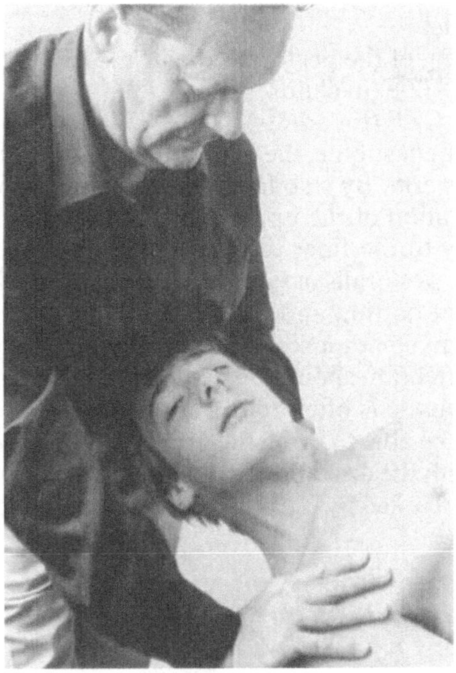

Fig. 113

Spinal Area: Upper and mid-thoracic spine

Type of Examination: Testing for muscles that hold the shoulder blade in place (rhomboid muscle, horizontal and descending portions of the trapezius muscle, serratus anterior muscle).

Diagnostic Usefulness: Moderate: CZE, SWI

Procedure: The patient is prone with his hands under the abdomen so that the scapulae are pulled anteriorly and laterally. In a vise-like grip, the examiner's thumb and a commissure, that is formed by fingers one and two and the radial edge of the index finger, the operator moves medially under the inferior angle of the scapula. The operator's hands are crossed over the patient's back and fix both scapulae (Fig. 114). The patient is now asked to move the scapula medially and inferiorly. Compared are muscle strength on both sides.

Remarks: Often weakening in the muscles responsible for holding the shoulder blade to the thorax is found.

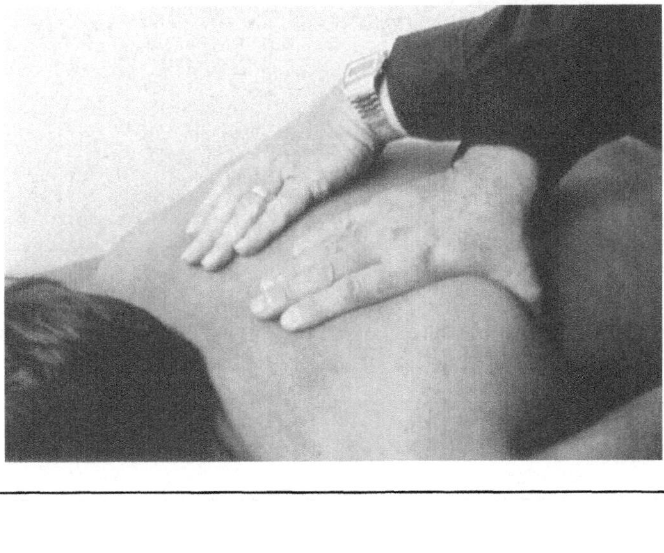

Fig. 114

Spinal Area: Thoracic Inlet

Type of Examination: Length testing of the pectoralis major muscle.

Diagnostic Usefulness: Great: CZE (in children)
Moderate: CZE (for adults), DEN, SWI

Procedure: With the patient supine, the operator abducts, externally rotates and elevates the patient's arm. By stabilizing the sternum with his full arm, the operator prevents rotation of the upper part of the body. The operator palpates perpendicularly to the fiber direction with the same hand the individual segments of the pectoralis major muscle, consisting of the clavicular portion, the upper sternal portion and the lower sternal portion. The operator searches for painful myotendinoses in these individual muscle portions (Fig. 115).
Particular attention should be paid to the mid sternal portion, since shortening of the muscle is often found at the level of the second intercostal space. One should be able to bring the arm into a horizontal position without causing pain. With the arm abducted, elevated and externally rotated, the examination is concluded by introducing slight stretch to the pectoralis major muscle.

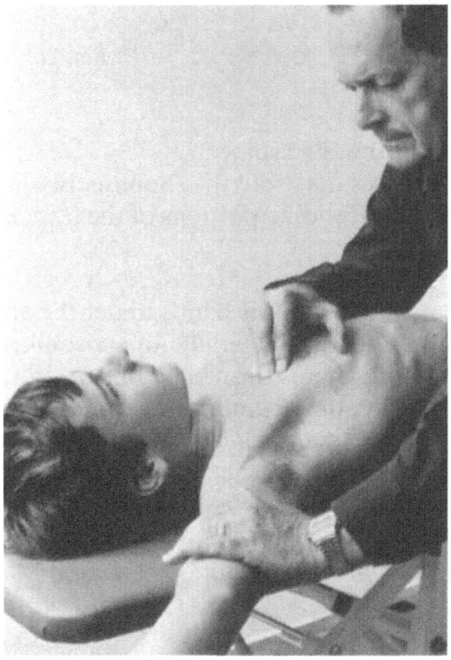

Fig. 115

Spinal Area: Upper and mid-thoracic spine

Type of Examination: Evaluation of muscles responsible for stabilizing the shoulder blade (i.e., serratus anterior muscle).

Diagnostic Usefulness: Great: CZE
Moderate: SWI

Procedure: The patient is prone with the arms and hands resting at his side on the examination table. The patient then pushes himself up from the table ("push-up types" of motion, Fig. 116). The patient should be in a well extended position (if the patient is too weak to perform this maneuver, he or she can start from a kneechest position).
This procedure evaluates the position of both scapulae. If there is weakning on one side the medial border of the scapula on that side is seen to form a step-like drop off. This difference becomes even more pronounced when the extended body returns to the normal prone position.

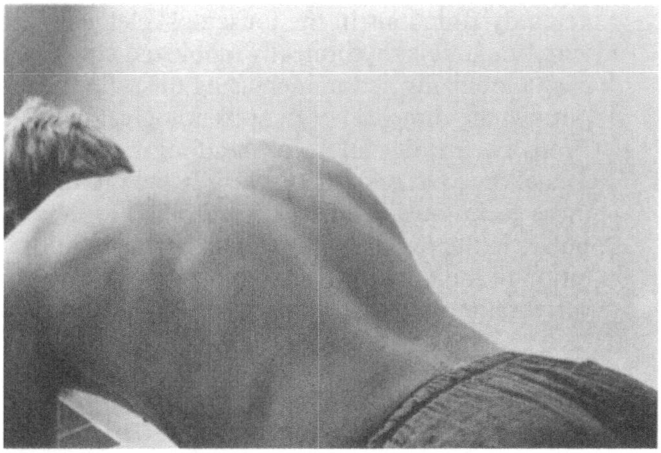

Fig. 116

4.3 Treatment

4.3.1 General Remarks Regarding Treatment Procedures

Even though there were differences in regard to frequency and specific details of the individual treatment procedures, the group came to general agreement regarding the major principles that underly the treatment techniques in manual medicine.
Presented here, in condensed form, are these differences concerning for the major considerations brought forth by the individual schools.
It was agreed that the individual treatment procedure should be classified according to one of the following two categories: 1) consisting of mobilizing techniques without impulse (thrust), 2) consisting of mobilizing techniques with impulse (thrust).

4.3.1.1 Mobilization Without Impulse (Thrust)

1. Muscle Energy (Inhibitory) Techniques

- The restricted barrier is engaged in three planes.
- A contact is applied for counterforce.

- The patient applies small isometric contraction against the counter-force as directed by the operator.
- The amount of force applied by the patient depends on:
  - the localized hyperirritability of a part of the muscle (minimal force),
  - total muscle irritability (greater force),
  - total muscle irritability and palpable connective tissue changes (chronic pain) as seen with maximum isometric muscle contraction.

After the isometric contraction, which lasts between 7 and 12 seconds, the involved muscles or the functionally abnormal joints are stretched or mobilized in the direction of the physiological barrier.

2. Articulatory Techniques (Joint Mobilization)

Articulatory techniques are primarily used when the patient presents with acute dysfunctions in the musculoskeletal system. The hypomobile joint or vertebral unit is rhythmically mobilized along its three planes of motion with each mobilizing action increasing the range of motion of the adjoining bony parts in the direction of the physiological barrier.
From a neurophysiological standpoint, one assumes that the mechanoreceptors of the joint capsule (especially the rapidly adapting) are stimualted with these techniques leading to pre-synaptic inhibition of the nociceptive impulses in the region of the dorsal horns. In addition to the pre-synaptic inhibition of the nociceptive afferent impulses, one could imagine that the paravertebral muscles are reflexogenically influenced.

4.3.1.2 Mobilization with Impulse (Thrust)

- The restrictive barrier of the involved joint is engaged in three planes.
- The operator stabilizes both the distal and proximal spinae segments ("locking" of such).
- The operator has the patient relax completely, and at the end of expiration introduces a high velocity, low amplitude thrust in the painfree direction.
- When applying mobilization with impulse, the following four factors are of primary importance: the joints must be in the correct position, the distal and proximal vertebral units are to be fixed, complete patient relaxation, manipulation in the painfree direction of the restricted barrier.

4.3.1.3 Therapeutic Guidelines and Sequence in the Individual Schools

USA, CZE, SWI, and FRG:
- In patients with chronic dysfunctions, one attempts to restore joint function to normal by the use of mobilization without impulse. For patients with acute dysfunctions one chooses mobilization with impulse.
- Stretching of shortened muscles.
- Strengthening of weak muscles.
- Correction of sterotypic motion patterns (coordination, activities of daily living), home training.

Denmark:
- Passive soft tissue treatment of the painful regions (rhythmic muscle massage, infiltration of muscle insertions, ligaments).
- Traction of the affected vertebral segment or regions according to the anatomy of the axial skeleton.
- Articulation without impulse (thrust).
- Articulation (manipulation) with impulse (thrust).
- Treatment for muscular imbalance (stretching of shortened and strengthening of weakened muscles).
- Exercise and training of sterotypic motion patterns encountered in daily living (Back School).

United Kingdom:
- Patient relaxation including psychological relaxation.
- Mobilization with impulse (thrust) (manipulation).
- Muscle stretch techniques (generally unspecific).
- Practical instructions to the patient for improvement of posture and stereotypic motion patterns (initially in conjunction with physiotherapy, later alone in home training).
- Back School (in conjunction with physiotherapist in a group).

4.3.2 Mobilization Without Impulse (No Thrust)

Type of Treatment: Mobilization without impulse
Goal: Nonspecific improvement of motion in the segments C3–C4 to T4–T5
Treatment Technique: Traction
Therapeutic Usefulness: Great: DEN
Moderate: SWI, UK
Little: FRG

Procedure: The patient is sitting. The thenar eminence of both hands is placed under the mastoid processes and, with the cervical spine slightly flexed, rhythmic traction motions are performed. The elbows are carried freely and do not come to rest on the patient's shoulders (Fig. 117). A variation with the patient in the supine position is shown in Figure 118.

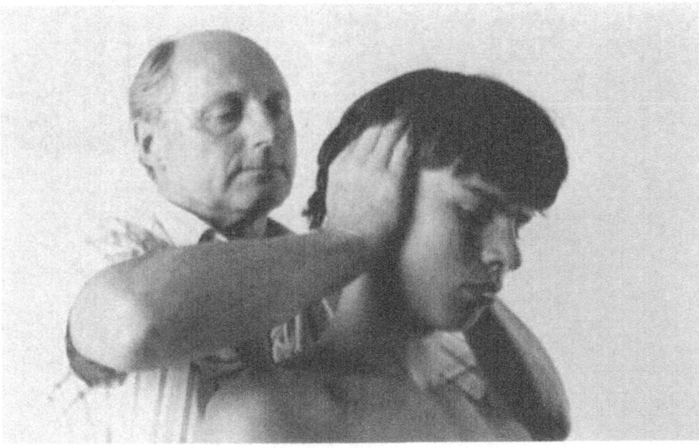

Fig. 117

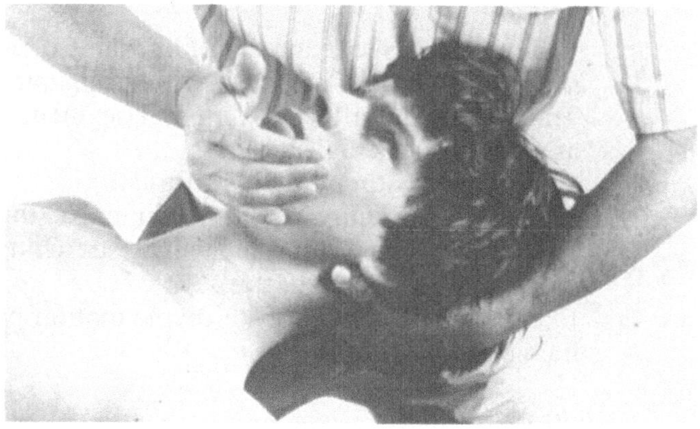

Fig. 118

Type of Treatment: Mobilization with/without impulse
Goal: Improvement of lateral sidebending and flexion the upper thoracic spine.
Treatment Technique: Mobilization or manipulation techniques for rotation and sidebending

Therapeutic Usefulness: Great: USA, DEN
Moderate: CZE

Procedure: For example, the patient is in the left side lying position. The operator's left thumb rests over the spinous process of T2 in this case. The patient's head rests on the operator's hand and forearm (Fig. 119).

Starting with this position, one can establish treatment using either mobilization procedures (including the application of post-isometric relaxation) or manipulation procedures. The thrusting force, in this case, is supplied through the right hand.

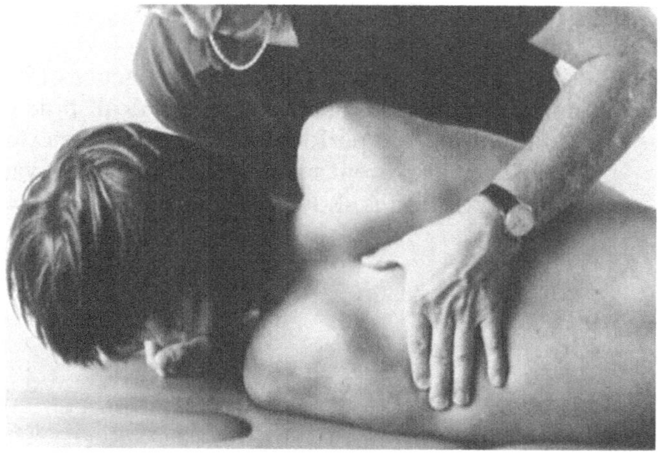

Fig. 119

Type of Treatment: Mobilization with or without impulse

Goal: Improvement of rotation, flexion and sidebending motions in the lower cervical spine.

Treatment Technique: Manipulation techniques for rotation and sidebending

Therapeutic Usefulness: Great: SWI, UK, CZE
Moderate: FRG, DEN

Procedure: The patient is sitting upright while the operator stands at the patient's side (in this example at the patient's right side). Using a vice-like grip applied to the spinous process and the vertebral arch, C5, for instance, is immobilized. In this case, the operator's ulnar border of the right small finger rests on the vertebral arch of C4 (Fig. 120).
The impulse consists of flexion, rotation (right) and sidebending (right) components.

Remarks: This technique can also be carried out with the patient supine (Fig. 121). Mobilization techniques without impulse can also easily be applied as can post-isometric relaxation techniques.

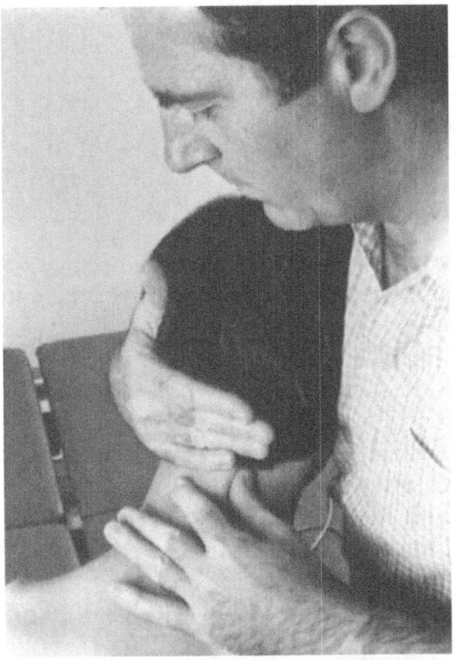

Fig. 120

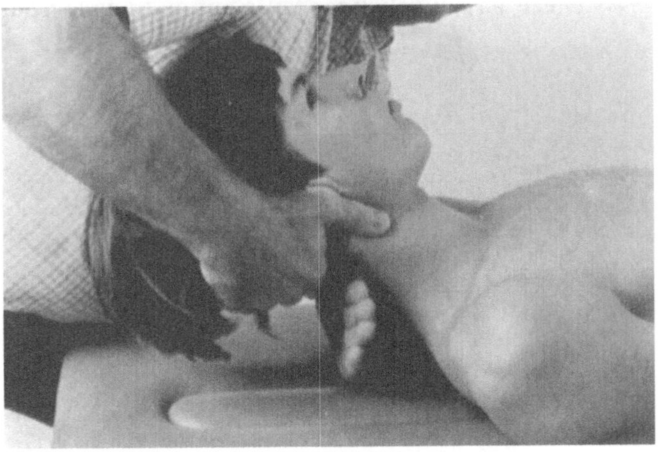

Fig. 121

4.3.3 Mobilization With Impulse (Thrust Techniques)

Type of Treatment: Mobilization with impulse
Goal: General improvement of motion in the lower cervical spine.
Type of Technique: Manipulation with traction
Therapeutic Usefulness: Great: SWI
Little: FRG
Procedure: The patient is supine. The cervical spine is slightly extended and somewhat sidebent towards the operator. The proximal phalanx of the thrusting hand lies dorso-laterally on C4, for instance. The impulse is in a superior direction (Fig. 122).

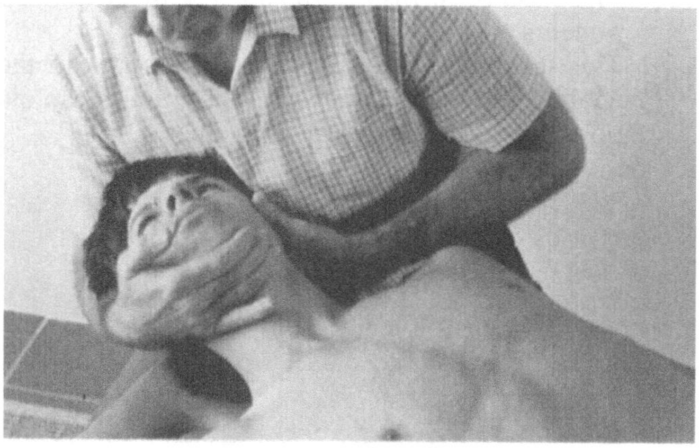

Fig. 122

Type of Treatment: Mobilization with impulse
Goal: Improvement of flexion in the cervico-thoracic junction.
Type of Technique: Manipulation for flexion motion
Therapeutic Usefulness: Great: DEN
Moderate: UK
Little: FRG
Procedure: The patient, who is sitting, reaches with both hands behind the neck. The operator reaches around the patient's upper arms and also embraces the patient's neck with his hands. The operator's fingers are then placed over the proximal spinous processes of those vertebral units that will be manipulated (Fig. 123).
Manipulation is then carried out with both hands using thrust with sudden traction and flexion.
Remarks: This is a relatively unspecific but quite dangerous technique.

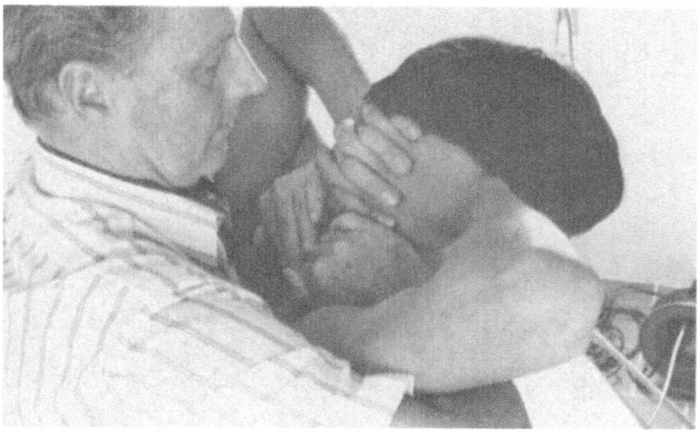

Fig. 123

Type of Treatment Mobilization with impulse
Goal: Improvement of rotation, sidebending, and extension in the upper thoracic spine.
Type of Technique: Manipulation for extention and sidebending
Therapeutic Usefulness: Great: DEN, USA, CZE, UK, FRG
Procedure: The patient is supine, with his arms crossed in front (the left arm, for example, rests anteriorly). Using his left hand, the operator rotates the patient's upper body towards himself by lifting the patient's left shoulder (Fig. 224). The operator's right thenar eminence is then placed over the left transverse process of, in this case, T1–C7, and patient is rotated back to the normal supine position. Those vertebral units that will be manipulated are brought into slight flexion (Fig. 125). The operator's body comes to rest on the patient's elbow and introduces some further stretch in this flexed position. He then allows the patient's upper body to move backward and introduces then left sidebending as well as extension (superiorly and in the thoracic region to the left).

The impulse in the direction of T1 and T2 is effected through the operator's body leaning on the patient's elbows.

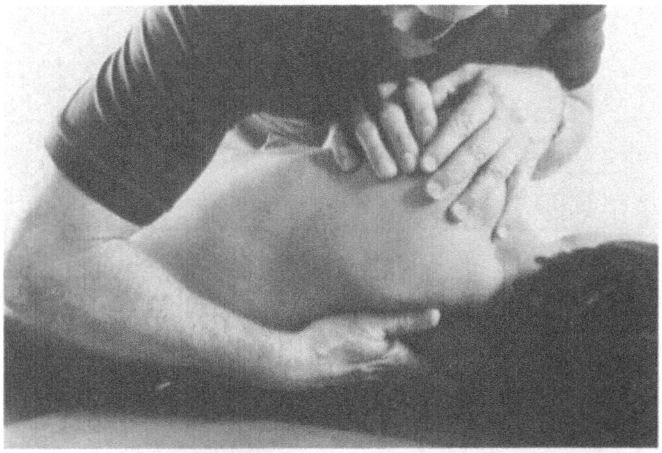

Fig. 124

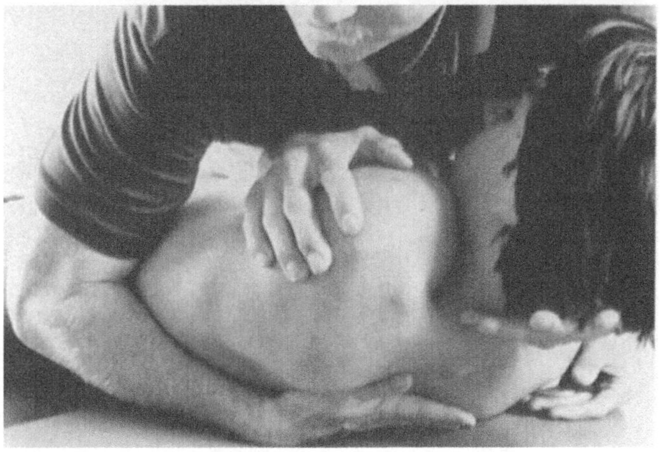

Fig. 125

Type of Treatment: Mobilization with impulse
Goal: Improvement of sidebending, rotation, and extension (T1–T2).
Type of Technique: Manipulation for extension, rotation and sidebending

Therapeutic Usefulness: Great: SWI, CZE, USA

Procedure: The patient is prone. The operator stands at the side of the patient (in this example, the left side). The operator's (right) ulnar hand border makes contact with articular process of T2, for example.

In this example, the cervical spine is rotated to the left and sidebent to the right, while the thoraco-cervical junction is flexed. The left hand of the operator stabilizes the temporaloccipital region (Fig. 126). Figures 127, 128, demonstrate variations presented by the Swiss and American schools, respectively.

The impulse follows the direction of rotation (in this example on T2) with simultaneous traction exerted on the total cervical spine provided by the left hand.

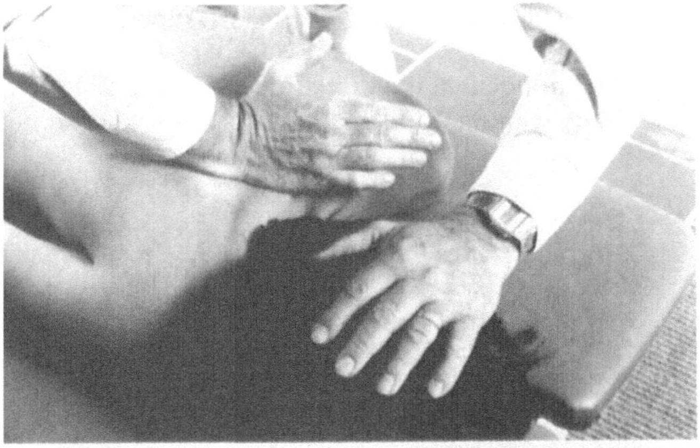

Fig. 126

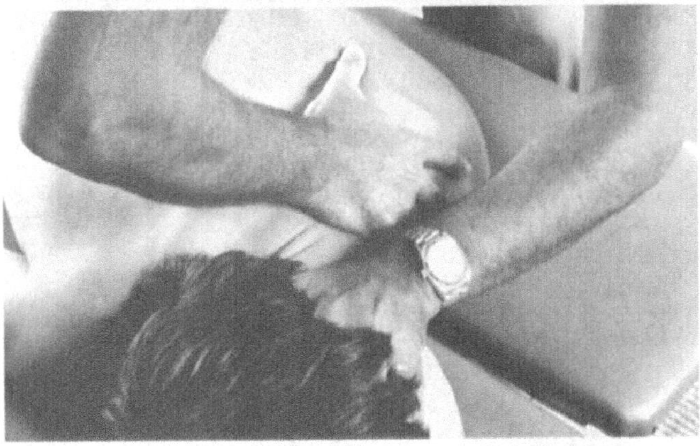

Fig. 127

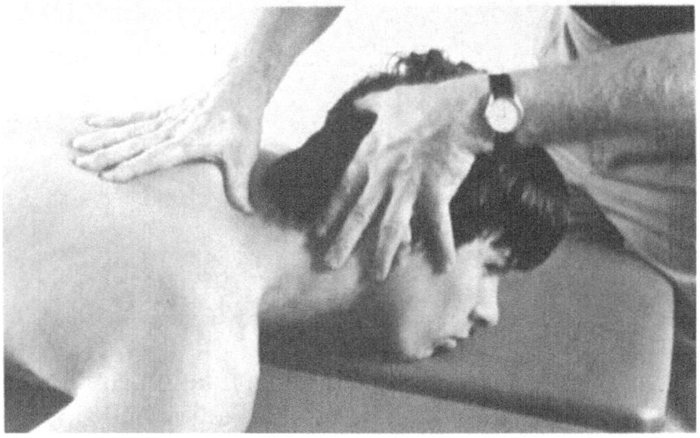

Fig. 128

Type of Treatment: Mobilization with impulse
Goal: Improvement of rotation motion in the lower cervical spine.
Type of Technique: Manipulation for rotation
Therapeutic Usefulness: Great: DEN, UK
Procedure: The patient is supine and rests his head on the forearm of the operator (i.e., the right forearm) whose hand cradles the patient's chin. The second metacarpal phalangeal joint of the right hand makes bony contact with the articular process of C4 for example (Fig. 129). The impulse is provided by the left hand and is directed to the right.

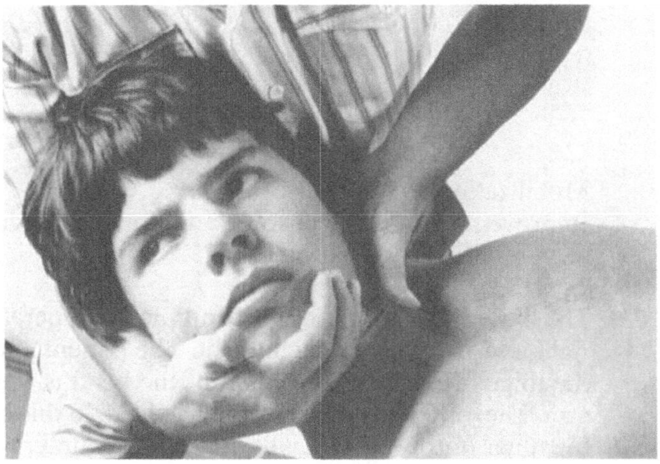

Fig. 129

Type of Treatment: Mobilization with impulse
Goal: Improvement of cervical spine rotation.
Type of Technique: Manipulation for rotation
Therapeutic Usefulness: Great: SWI, FRG
Moderate: DEN, CZE, UK
Procedure: The patient is sitting. The operator, who is close to the patient, palpates with the left middle finger, for instance, the spinous process of C4 while the right hand introduces sidebending to the barrier (Fig. 130) accompanied by slight rotation to the left.
The impulse is provided by the middle finger resting on the joint (C4) and is directed along left rotation (Fig. 131).

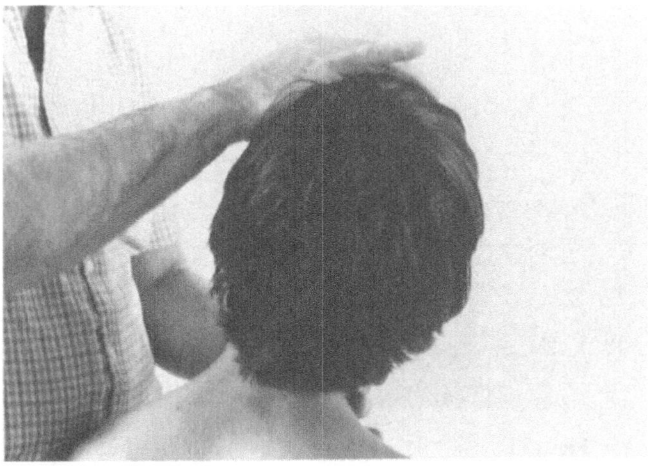

Fig. 130

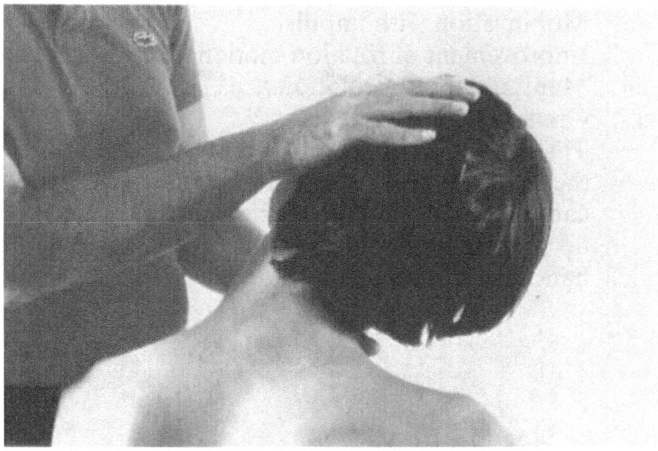

Fig. 131

Type of Treatment: Mobilization with impulse
Goal: Improvement of cervical spine and upper thoracic rotation.
Type of Technique: Manipulation for rotation
Therapeutic Usefulness: Great: DEN, SWI
Procedure: The patient is sitting. In this example, the operator stands somewhat to the right and posterior to the patient. The patient's right arm is positioned over the thigh. The temporal region of the head is stabilized with the right forearm. The joint and spinous process of C4, in this example, are stabilized with the ulnar border of the right hand. The counter force is applied at the distal spinous process of C5 with the left thumb (Figs. 132, 133).
The impulse is provided by the left thumb, while simultaneous rotation, slight sidebending and traction of the head with the right forearm and hand are introduced.

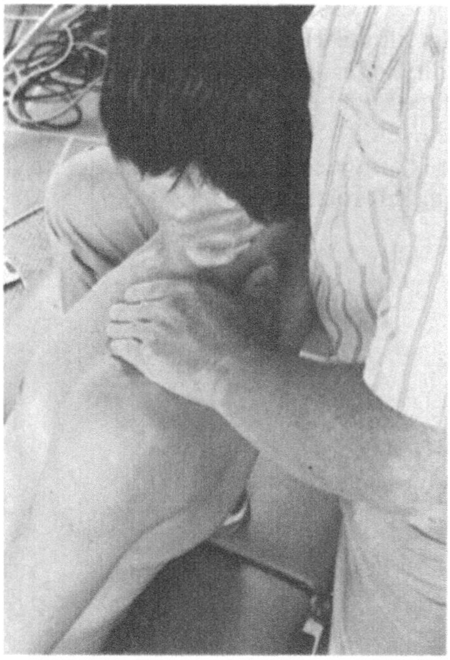

Fig. 132

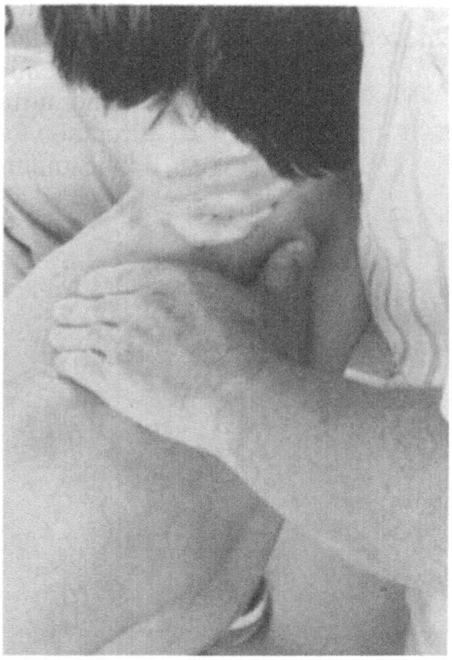

Fig. 133

Type of Treatment:	Mobilization with impulse
Goal:	Improvement of mid and lower cervical spine rotation.
Type of Technique:	Manipulation for rotation
Therapeutic Usefulness:	Great: SWI, DEN Moderate: CZE Little: FRG
Procedure:	The patient is supine. In this example, the operator's second metacarpal-phalangeal joint of the left hand makes contact with the posterior portion of the articular process of the vertebra (C4, in this case). The other hand (right) cradles the chin and exerts slight traction (Fig. 134). The impulse is provided by the operator's left hand and is directed along the rotation motion (right) (Fig. 135).
Remarks:	This manipulative procedure is directed towards the joint on the restricted side.

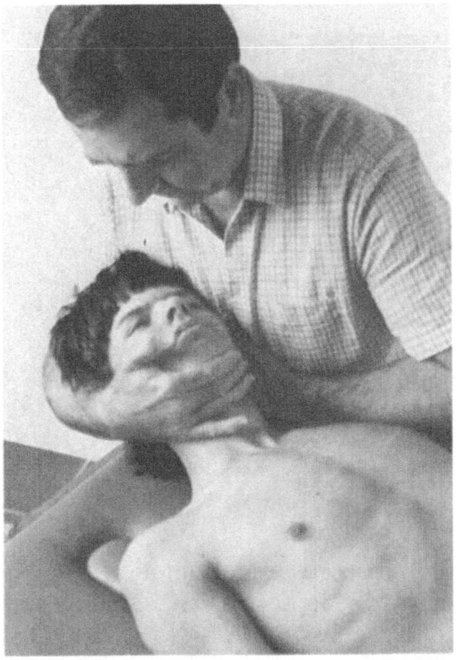

Fig. 134

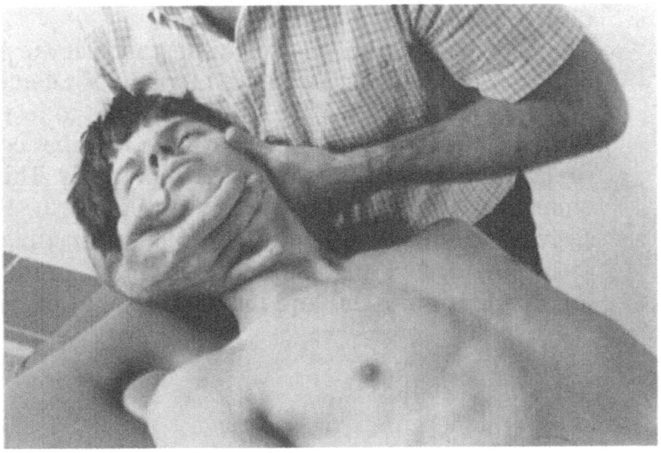

Fig. 135

Type of Treatment: Mobilization utilizing respiratory motion
Goal: Improvement of rib mobility during expiration.
Type of Technique: Rib mobilization
Therapeutic Usefulness: Great: USA,FRG
Procedure: The patient is supine. The operator stands laterally behind the patient's head. The operator's thumb is placed at the superior border and on the anterior portion of the rib that resists exhalation. With his other hand, the operator flexes and sidebends the thoracic spine to the level of the resisting rib on the same side. The patient is then instructed to exhale (Fig. 136). The operator's fingers fellow the exhalation motion of the rib, holding the ribs in the final exhalation position. The patient is then asked to slightly inhale and again to deeply exhale, whereby the operator's hand follows the expiratory motion. This is repeated three to four times. The patient's spine is then brought back into the neutral position with the thumbs, however, holding the rib in its expiratory position. The soft tissues are thus stretched.

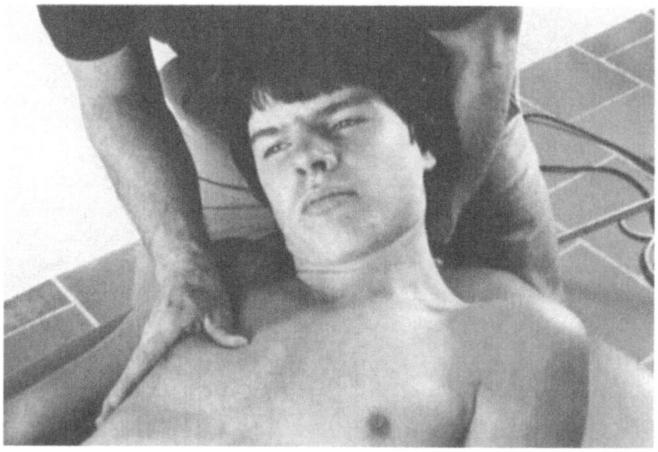

Fig. 136

Type of Treatment: Mobilization utilizing respiratory motion
Goal: Improvement of rib motion when resisting inspiration ("stuck in expiration").
Type of Technique: Rib mobilization
Therapeutic Usefulness: Great: USA, FRG
Procedure: The patient is supine. The operator stands at the patient's side. The patient's arm is maximally elevated and internally rotated in the shoulder joint of the affected side, such that the forearm comes to rest on the patient's forehead. With his/her middle finger, the operator makes contact with the angle of the rib laterally pulling the same latero-inferiorly. The opposite hand provides a counterforce at the elbow of the elevated arm (Fig. 137). The patient is instructed to inhale and simultaneously push the elbow against the counter force provided by the operator. This effects contraction of the pectoralis major and minor muscles and introduces superior movement of the ribs.

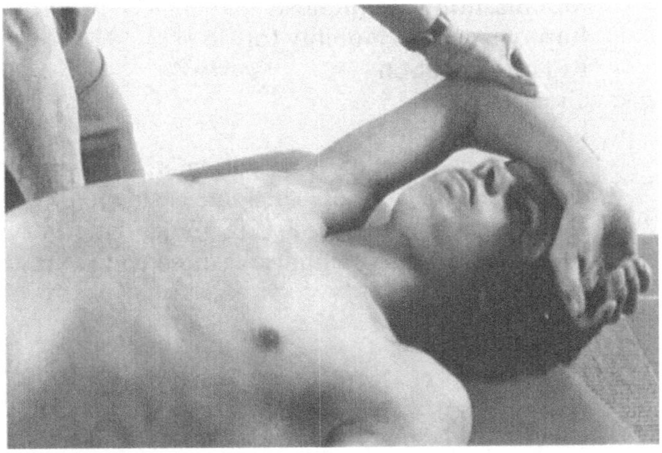

Fig. 137

Type of Treatment: Mobilization with impulse
Goal: Improvement of rib I mobility
Type of Technique: Rib manipulation
Therapeutic Usefulness: Moderate: FRG
Procedure: The patient is supine. The patient's head rests on the tip of the chin and the cervical spine is rotated to one side (i.e., left). The operator then stabilizes the patient's head with his/her right hand in this example. Contact is made at the angle of the first rib with the pisiform bone (Fig. 138).
In this example, the impulse is provided through the pisiform bone of the left hand with the force being directed toward the left acromio-clavicular joint.

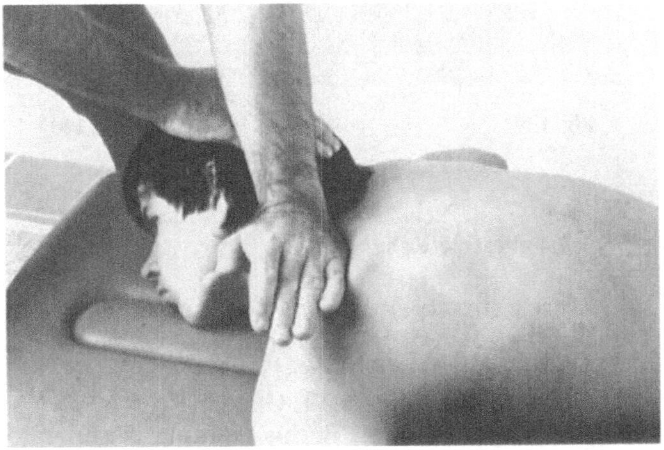

Fig. 138

Type of Treatment: Mobilization with impulse
Goal: Improvement of mobility for rib I
Type of Technique: Rib manipulation
Therapeutic Usefulness: Great: SWI
Little: FRG
Procedure: The patient is sitting. The patient's left arm is draped over the operator's flexed left leg. The cervical spine is sidebent. The operator's right index finger is placed on the first rib (Fig. 139). Figure 140 shows the German variation. In this example, the impulse is directed toward the left hip of the patient.

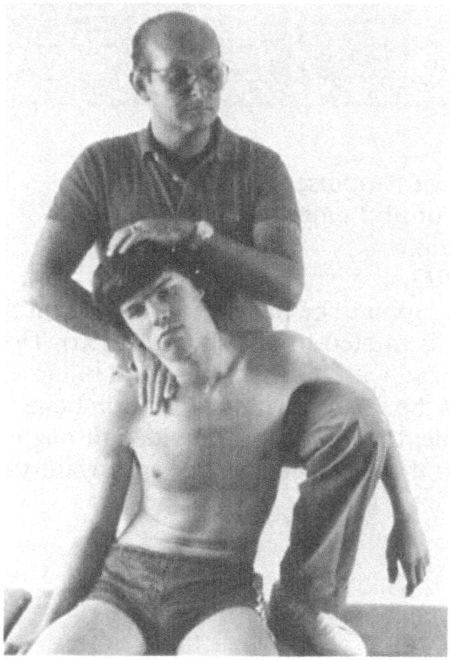

Fig. 139

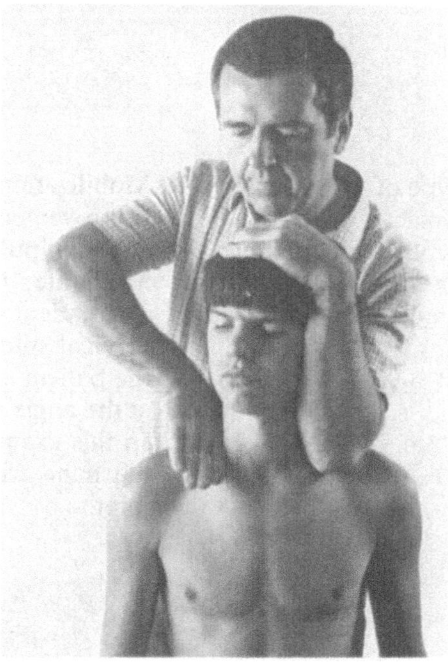

Fig. 140

4.3.4 Muscle Rehabilitation

Type of Treatment: Muscle stretching utilizing post-isometric relaxation
Goal: Improvement of rotation at the C4–C5 segment
Type of Technique: Muscle stretch techniques
Therapeutic Usefulness: Great: FRG, USA, SWI, UK, CZE
Procedure: The patient is sitting. In this example, the operator stands to the right side of the patient. The operator's right middle finger establishes contact with the articular process of C5. The left hand provides an isometric counterforce at the patient's mid-forehead. The vertebral column, in this example, is both maximally rotated and sidebent to the left (Fig. 141).
The patient tries to rotate and sidebend his forehead to the right against the operator's counterforce by isometrically contracting the muscles.

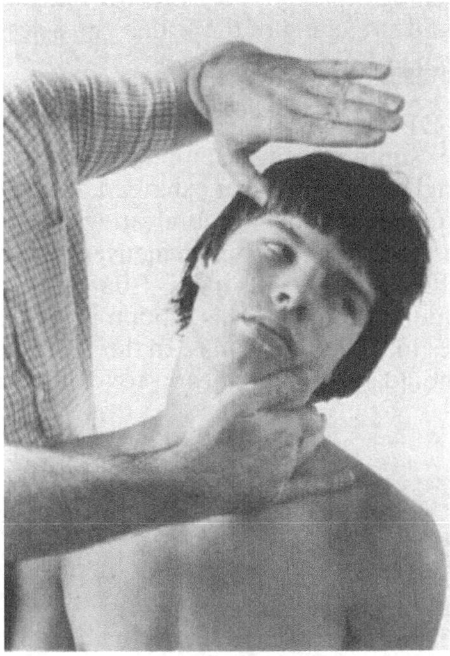

Fig. 141

Type of Treatment:	Muscle stretching utilizing post-isometric relaxation
Goal:	Lengthening of the levator scapulae muscle (i. e., on the right side)
Type of Technique:	Muscle stretch technique
Therapeutic Usefulness:	Great: SWI, FRG, CZE
	Moderate: DEN
	Little: USA
Procedure:	The patient is supine. In this example, the cervical spine is flexed, rotated to the left and sidebent slightly to the left. The patient's right arm is maximally elevated and externally rotated in the shoulder joint. The patient's hand is placed under the head, while his right elbow finds support on the operator's body. The patient then isometrically contracts the muscles with the right arm in the direction of the operator (Fig. 142). During the relaxation phase, the operator pushes the patient's upper arm inferiorly. Due to the close packed scapulo-humeral joint, the scapula is translated inferiorly.

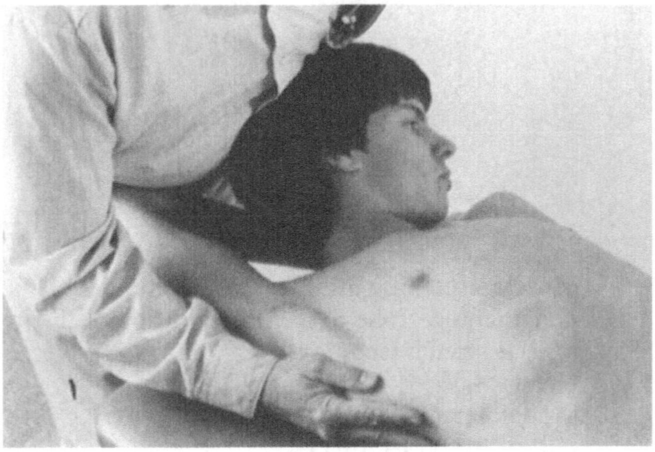

Fig. 142

Type of Treatment: Muscle stretching utilizing post-isometric relaxation
Goal: Relaxation and stretching of the scalene muscles
Type of Technique: Muscle stretch technique
Therapeutic Usefulness: Great: CZE
Moderate: DEN

Procedure: The patient is supine. In this example, the cervical spine is rotated and side-bent to the right and somewhat extended. In the extended and rotated positions, compression of the vertebral artery is most likely, and one should therefore be careful during this maneuver. The cervico-thoracic junction is fixed with the operator's left hand. Isometric rotation to the left and side-bending to the left follows. This motion is controlled by having the patient move his eyes to the left (Fig. 143). In the postisometric relaxation phase, the eyes' gaze should be straight ahead, stretching (Fig. 144).

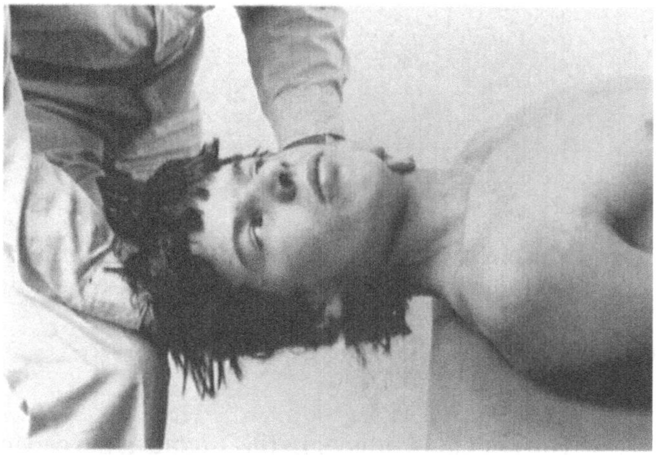

Fig. 143

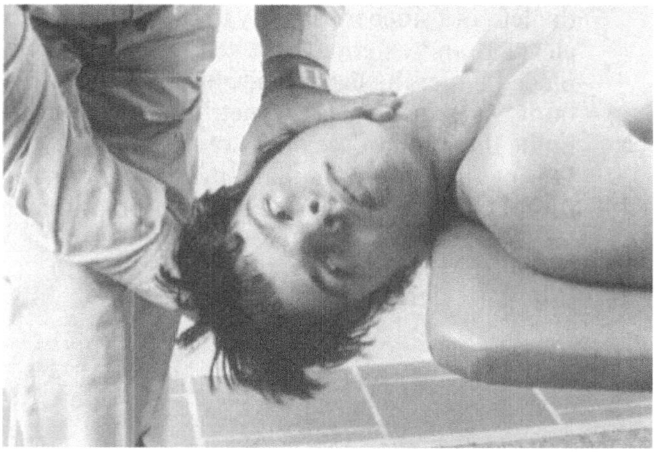

Fig. 144

Type of Treatment: Muscle stretching utilizing post-isometric relaxation
Goal: Lengthening of the descending portion of the trapezius muscle
Type of Technique: Muscle stretch technique
Therapeutic Usefulness: Great:
Moderate: CZE, SWI, DEN
Little: USA, FRG

Procedure: The patient is supine. In this example, the cervical spine is flexed and somewhat rotated to the right and sidebent to the left. The operator's left hand, in this case, as well as the whole body protect the patient's head. The operator's right hand provides the counterforce on the patient's right shoulder (Fig. 145).
Isometric contraction of the shoulder muscles is against the operator's counterforce (i. e., his right hand).
During the relaxation period the operator pushes the patient's shoulder inferiorly.

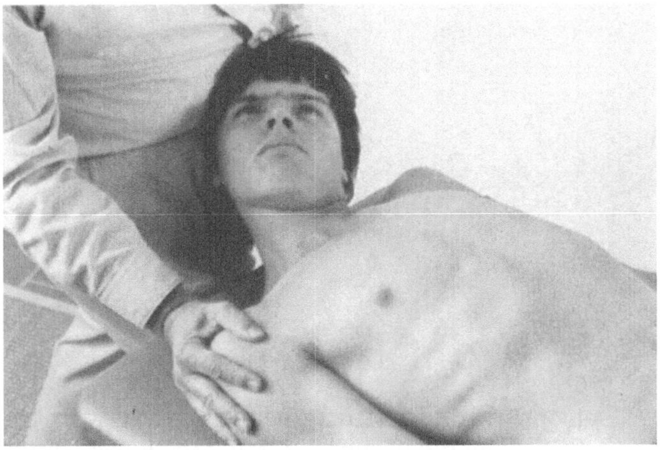

Fig. 145

Type of Treatment: Muscle stretching utilizing post-iosmetric relaxation
Goal: Stretching of the sternocleidomastoid muscle
Type of Technique: Muscle stretch technique
Therapeutic Usefulness: Moderate: CZE
Little: USA, FRG, SWI, DEN

Procedure: The patient is supine. In this case the cervical spine is rotated 45° to the left and sidebent to the left as well. The operator's left hand secures the patient's hand. The counterforce is localized with the operator's right hand on the right side of the head (Fig. 146).
Isometric contraction of the sternocleidomastoid muscle lasts for 10 seconds. The muscle is stretched during the post-isometric relaxation period.

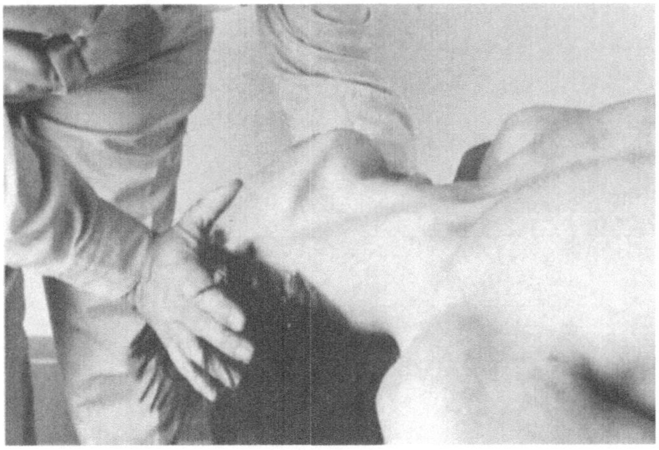

Fig. 146

Type of Treatment: Isometric muscle strengthening
Goal: Strengthening of the deep cervical spine flexor muscles
Type of Technique: Isometric muscle strength technique
Therapeutic Usefulness: Great: CZE, FRG, SWI
Procedure: The operator provides a counterforce to the patient's chin. The patient contracts his muscles isometrically along a flexioninclination direction (Fig. 147).

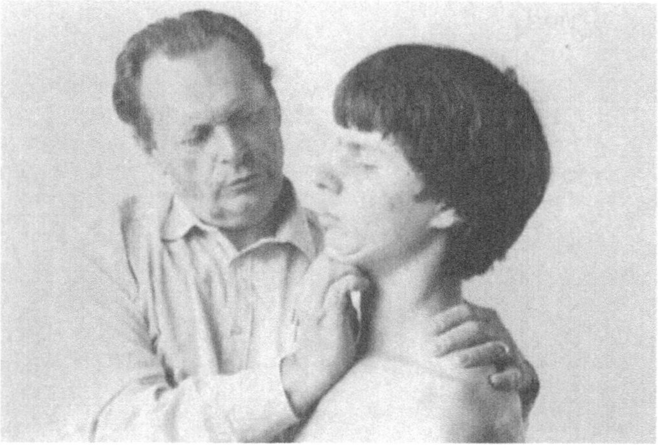

Fig. 147

Type of Treatment: Isometric muscle strengthening
Goal: Strengthening of muscles fixing the lower shoulder blade
Type of Technique: Isometric muscle strengthening
Therapeutic Usefulness: Great: CZE, SWI
Procedure: The patient is sitting in a chair that has a midhigh back support. The patient moves his shoulder blades toward the border of the back support and is requested to pull the shoulder blades infero-medially whereby the chair's back support provides the unyielding resistance (Fig. 148).

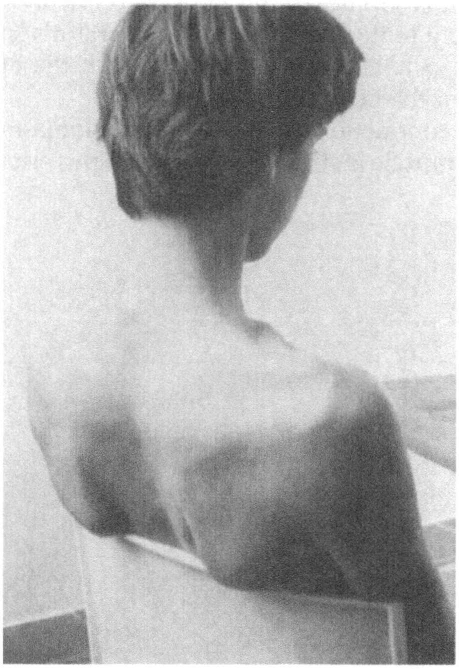

Fig. 148

4.4 Summary

The group's goal was to establish characteristics specific to the cervicothoracic junction. They include:
- The influence different muscles have on the function of the cervicothoracic junction. This is the result of the functional relationship of the cervicothoracic junction in regard to the head, the shoulder girdle, the entire vertebral column and the pelvis. Special consideration must be given here to the function of the longissimus cervicis and capitis muscles, the iliocostalis muscle and the semispinalis capitis muscle.
- The cervico-thoracic junction and its relation to the function of the thorax, the respiratory movements, and the upper extremities.
- The special consideration regarding the influence of the autonomic nervous system on this region.
- The influence of psychogenic factors on the function of the cervicothoracic junction as well as the great amounts of loading and strain on this section of the vertebral column as a result of daily activities.
- The influence on this region resulting from wrong body posture, especially seen in persons who sit a lot.

Since it is difficult to establish a differential diagnosis of pathogenesis for the cervico-thoracic junction, a very careful approach is necessary:
- A single symptom does not tell us much and cannot give any indication for the cause.
- A Complete case history and a general physical examination of the patient will improve the understanding of pathogenic correlations.
- Even if a certain pattern of pathological findings have been established conclusions cannot be automatically drawn (caveat: viscero-somatic reflexes).

Three findings must be differentiated when diagnosing segmental dysfunction:
- Soft tissue changes,
- Articular changes,
- Neuro-muscular changes.

Thus, one cannot be concerned with functional aspects of joint physiology only, but should also consider muscular balance as well as other influences on the musculature (such as reflex phenomena), that are caused by excessive stimulation of mechano- and nociceptors.
In the cervical spine region, one should always consider the possibility of problems caused by the vertebral artery. Provocative testing for the vertebral artery should always precede manual treatment at the cervical spine (de-Kleijn testing, rotation-reclination testing, Unterberger-Test, in different head positions). Doppler sonography of the vertebral artery may also provide valuable information about possible functional disturbances in the vertebral artery.

4.4.1 Diagnosis

There was general consensus regarding the following points:
- The importance of a careful, systematic history.
- The evaluation of posture and the general physical examination for the whole body.

- Specific examination of the apophyseal joints and the joints of the upper extremities, in all three planes (X-axis: flexion-extension, Y-axis: axial rotation, Z-axis: sidebending).
- Careful evaluation of soft tissue changes, changes in the muscular patterns or muscular imbalance with the upper extremities included.
- Evaluation of the thorac inlet as well as respiratory muscles.

There was more disagreement about the importance of individual diagnostic findings than the technical details of the diagnostic evaluation itself. The German school, for instance, places greater emphasis on articular dysfunction then it does on findings of soft tissue or muscular changes. The Swiss school, on the other hand, is interested in the finding of segmental zones of irritation and systematic myotendinoses that are seen as the reflexogenic consequence of a causative disturbance in the vertebral unit, and is less interested in the segmental articular disturbances in all three planes. The representatives from the Czechoslovakian and Austrian schools place their primary interest in changes of muscular balance and changes in motion-patterns. The American osteopathic physicians concentrate heavily on the palpatory examination for joint function and attribute significant consideration to translatory motion patterns in the individual segments. Muscle imbalance is normally not evaluated by the American School.

4.4.2 Treatment and Techniques

In regard to treatment procedures, there was concensus as follows:
- Joint function should be normalized first with the appropriate therapeutic technique.
- Treatment of tightened, short muscles consists of stretching techniques while weakened muscles are to be strengthened with the appropriate exercises.
- It should be noted that treating acute problems is only one aspect of the overall approach. That is, great emphasis is placed on procedures that concern themselves with the underlying problems and when applied act in a preventative manner.
- In this context of the preventative approach the patient should be educated about his motor performance to facilitate coping with the activities of daily living.

4.4.3 Disagreement

There was only disagreement in regard to the usefulness and the treatment of choice in certain conditions, such as deciding whether to choose soft tissue techniques, mobilization without thrust or manipulation.

Whereas, the American, Czechoslovakian, Swiss and German schools start treating with soft tissue procedures and mobilization without impulse (thrust), the British school prefers the classical manipulative porcedures, such as mobilization with impulse (thrust), as first choice of treatment.

There was general agreement in regard to technique and procedure of the individual treatment procedures.

Some of the procedures presented by the Americans, who routinely employ muscle energy techniques, for instance, were new to some of the European schools.

Chapter 5

Thoracic Spine, Thoraco-Lumbar Junction and Ribs

Participants:
Czechoslovakia (CZE):
K. Lewit
Finland (FIN):
K. Rebola
France (F):
A. Gourjon
Sweden (SWE):
F. Mildenberger
Switzerland (SWI):
E. Schwarz, H. Alder
USA: M. Beal
West Germany (FRG):
R. Geiger

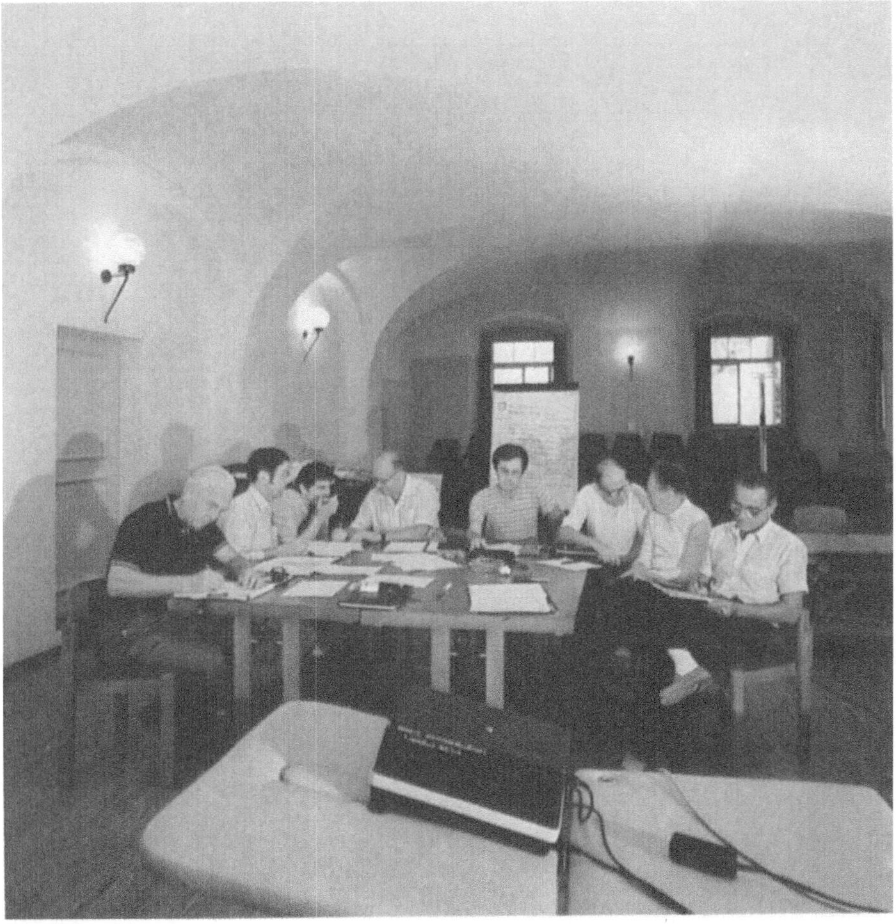

5.1 Biomechanics of the Thoracic Spine and Thoraco Lumbar Junction

The term mid-thoracic spine as used here includes the thoraco-lumbar junction and is defined as the region between the third thoracic vertebra (T3) and the second lumbar vertebra (L2). Inferiorly, this region includes the upper part of the lordotic curve of the lumbar spine while superiorly it is continuous with the kyphotic curve of the thoracic spine.
The biomechanical properties and range of motion of this area of the spine as well as the individual vertebrae are determined by the shape of the lumbar and thoracic spinal curves.
The articular surfaces of the thoracic vertebrae are inclined in two different planes, that is 60° about the X-axis and 20° about the Y-axis (Fig. 79).
Despite this double inclination of the joint surfaces, rotation is possible in all three planes (flexion-extension, sidebending and axial rotation).
Sidebending in the thoracic spine is accompanied by axial rotation (coupling patterns) (Fig. 149) similar to the cervical spine.

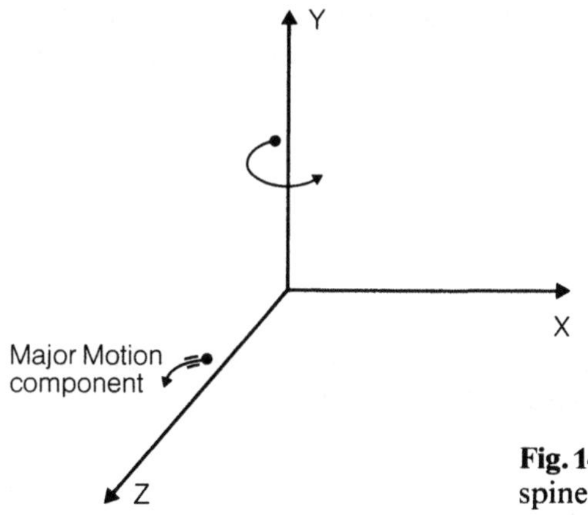

Fig. 149 Coupled motions seen with thoracic spine side bending

Axial rotation in the mid-thoracic spine is between 2°–8° and is coupled with sidebending measuring between 6°–8°. The thoraco-lumbar junction is the least mobile section in the thoracic spine.
The longitudinal ligament, the annulus fibrosus, the height of the intervertebral disc, the interspinous and supraspinous ligaments and the positions of the spinous processes all contribute to the small range of motion that is seen in the thoracic vertebra.
Significant stablization of the thoracic spine results from the ribs connecting the thoracic spine to the sternum. The thoracic spine is the longest portion of the spine. Further stability of the paired costovertebral and costotransverse joints is effected by a strong ligamentous apparatus.
The relatively rigid interconnection of the sternum and thoracic spine by the ribs gives the vertebral column tremendous stability against rotatory traumatic stress.
According to biomechanical calculations, the trunk can undergo a rotation of about 25° in the lower thoracic spine. Rotation is possible in this portion of the spine since the free ribs are unable to limit the rotational movement.
Transitional vertebrae such as those occurring at the thoraco-lumbar junction are of clinical importance. Frequently the 12th thoracic vertebra has superior articular processes which are identical to the thoracic articular pro-

cesses, whereas the inferior articular processes resemble those of a lumbar vertebra. The biomechanical action of T12 results from the different inclinations of the articular surfaces.
The mid thoracic spine at T4 and T5 is another transitional area. Kinesiological studies show that rotation in the cervical spine is often transmitted down to the third and fourth thoracic vertebrae. Clinical experience shows that this spinal area often presents with segmental dysfunctions. The fact that the strong fibers of the longissimus dorsi muscle insert at the transverse processes of T4 and T5 is significant. Also the strongest fibers of the semispinalis capitis muscle originate from the proximal portions of the transverse processes of T4 and T5. Thus, it could be assumed that even minimal functional disturbances in these muscles influence the biomechanics in this transitional area.
In addition to these two muscles which are representatives of the longissimus and the transversospinous system, the following muscles are also important in the thoracic spine and thoraco-lumbar junction: psoas major muscle, quadratus lumborum muscle, iliocostalis muscle, internal and external oblique muscles, and rectus abdominis muscle.
The respiratory movements and diaphragm function are also of special significance.

5.2 Diagnosis

5.2.1 Diagnostic Criteria Regarding the Thoracic Spine and the Thoraco-Lumbar Junction

Inspection

This includes the evaluation of overall thorax shape, position and orientation of the scapulae, shape of the angles of the waist, respiratory excursion, arm length, iliac crest and anal folds.

Motion Testing

- Gross motion testing in three planes with the patient standing.
- Regional motion testing in three planes, actively and passively with the patient sitting.
- Segmental motion testing of the thoracic spine in three planes with the patient sitting routinely performed by the American osteopathic school. However, the French and Swiss schools do not include this segmental motion testing in their diagnostic workup.

Soft Tissue Examination

The American representatives examine their patient sitting, whereas the European schools prefer the patient prone.

1. Palpation (Layer Tissue – Palpation)

- Skin drag
- Kibler-Fold
- Segmental myotendinosis (segmental muscle tension)
- Tender-painful points at the periosteum of the spinous processes and angles of the ribs.
- Zones of irritation (Swiss nomenclature), "point articulaire post postérieur" (French nomenclature). The segmental zones of irritation, a term coined by the Swiss school, are found at three locations: in the region of the articular processes, the costotransverse joint and the costal angle. Of practical importance is the zone of irritation that is located over the transverse process due to its easy accessibility. Provocative testing for zones of irritation can be performed in this region as well.

2. Autonomic Skin Reactions

- These phenomena may be the result of viscero-somatic reflexes.

3. Pain Provocation

- Springing test
- "Pression lateral contraire" (French school).

4. Rib Palpation

- Costotransverse joints
- Palpation of the ribs during respiration movements.

5. Neuromuscular Correlations

- Palpation of the identification muscles (psoas major muscle, longissimus dorsi muscle, semispinalis capitis muscle, etc.)
- Functional examination of the primarily postural muscles (pectoralis major muscle, quadratus lumborum muscle, psoas major muscle, etc.)
- Functional examination of the phasic muscles that normally become the weakened muscle groups (the inferior muscles responsible for holding the scapula in place, abdominal muscles).

In diagnostic testing, the osteopathic schools attribute greater significance to segmental motion testing, whereas the Swiss and French schools prefer the palpatory examination of the painful, systematized myotendinoses, and the segmental points of irritation ("point articulaire postérieur").

5.2.2 Soft Tissue Examination

Spinal Area: Mid thoracic spine, lumbo-sacral junction
Type of Examination: Superficial skin palpation
Diagnostic Usefulness: Great: USA, CZE
Moderate: FRA, SWI, SWE
None: FRG
Procedure: The palpating finger employes light touch to examine the skin in the paravertebral region: temperature, skin moisture and trophic changes are evaluated (Fig. 150).

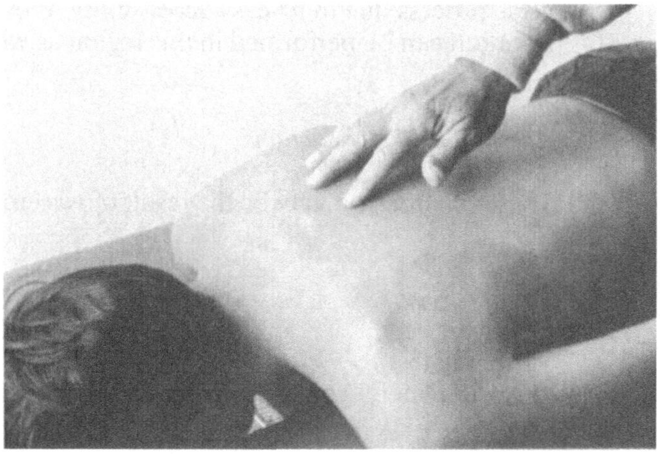

Fig. 150

Spinal Area: Entire vertebral column
Type of Examination: Subcutaneous tissue evaluation
Diagnostic Usefulness: Great: F
Moderate: SWE, SWI, CZE, FRG
None: USA
Procedure: Between his thumb and index finger, the examiner forms a skinfold ("Kibler-Fold," or "skin roll"). Evaluated are the mobility of the subcutaneous tissue in relation to the skin, adhesions and manifestations of pain (Fig. 151).

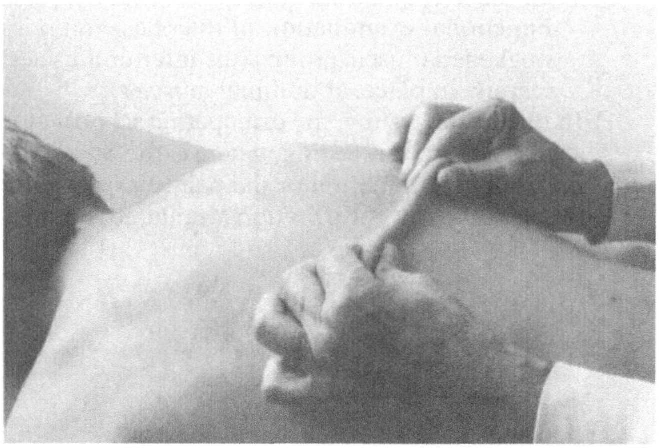

Fig. 151

Spinal Area: Entire vertebral column
Type of Examination: Gross palpatory evaluation of the paravertebral musculature
Diagnostic Usefulness: Great: CZE, USA, SWE, SWI, F
Moderate: FRG, F

Procedure: The palpating fingers are first placed over the spinous processes in the mid thoracic spine. The fingers are then moved over the paravertebral musculature so as to establish palpatory contact with the muscles (Fig. 152). Without trying to identify the individual muscle groups per se, one simply evaluates muscle tone, consistency and plasticity of the individual muscle bundles. During this examination procedure, attention is also paid to possible painful areas elicited during palpation.

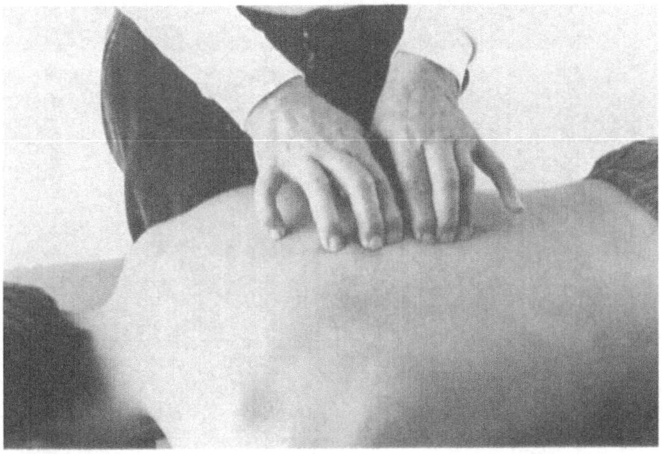

Fig. 152

Spinal Area: Entire vertebral column
Type of Examination: Indentification of bony landmarks, ligaments and apophyseal joints
Diagnostic Usefulness: Great: SWI, F
Moderate: USA, CZE, SWE, FRG

Procedure: The palpating finger identifies first the spinous process and then moves laterally and superiorly so as to reach the transverse processes and costal angles (Fig. 153).
This is followed by palpation of the segmental zones of irritation (SWI, Fig. 154), or the "point articulaire postérieur" (F). The French group applies lateral pressure against the spinous process to provoke pain, a maneuver called "pression latérale contraire."

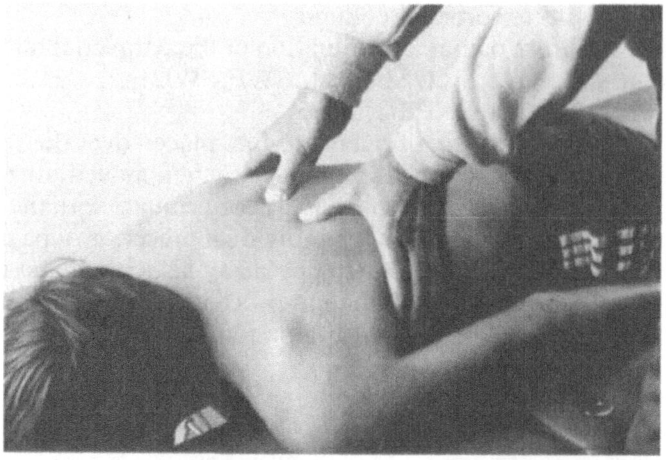

Fig. 153

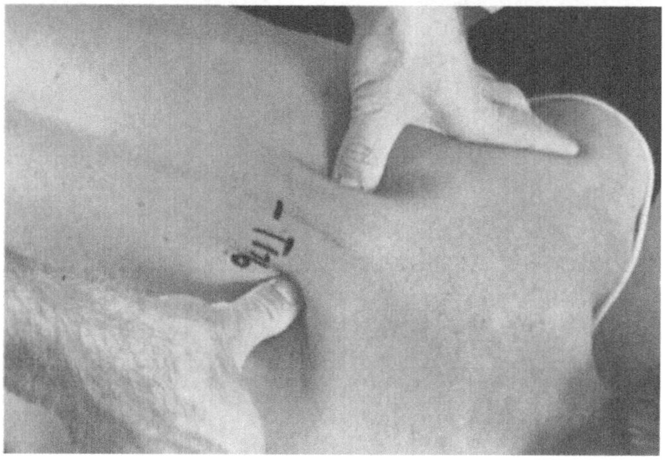

Fig. 154

5.2.3 Motion Testing

Spinal Area(s): Entire thoracic spine

Type of Examination: Segmental flexion and extension

Diagnostic Usefulness: Great: USA, SWE, CZE, FRG, F

Procedure: The operator stands at the side of the seated patient. American variation: the palpating thumb and index finger are placed on each side of the spinous process and then move inferiorly to the interspinous space. The examiner introduces passive maximum flexion and extension motions of the head with the other hand (Figs. 155, 156).

Check variation: the patient clasps his hands behind his neck while the examiner reaches around both of the patient's elbows introducing passive flexion and extension motions through the leverage of the subject's upper arms (Fig. 157). During this maneuver, segmental mobility of the spinous processes is evaluated.

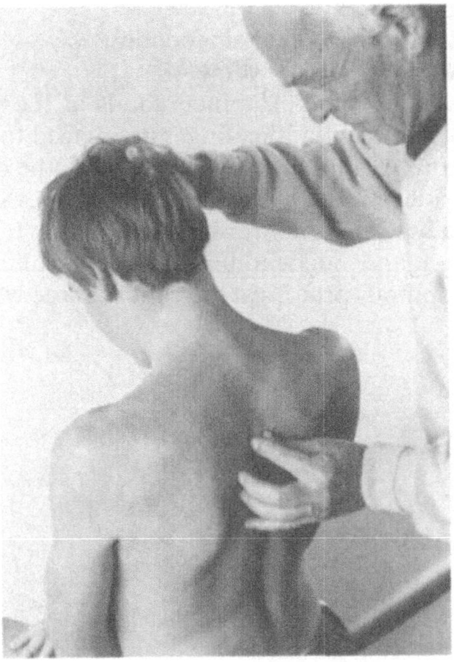

Fig. 155

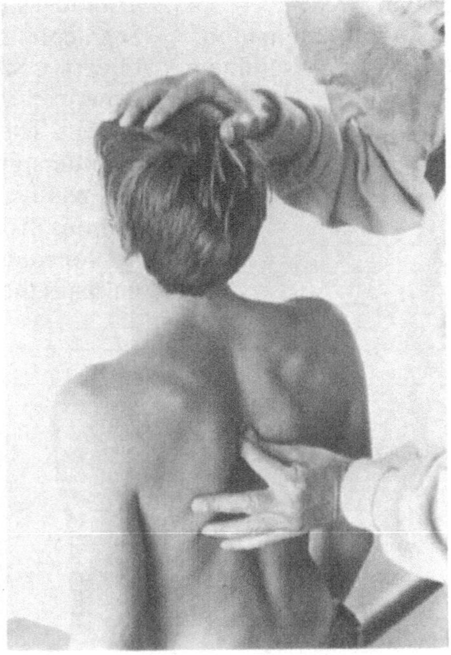

Fig. 156

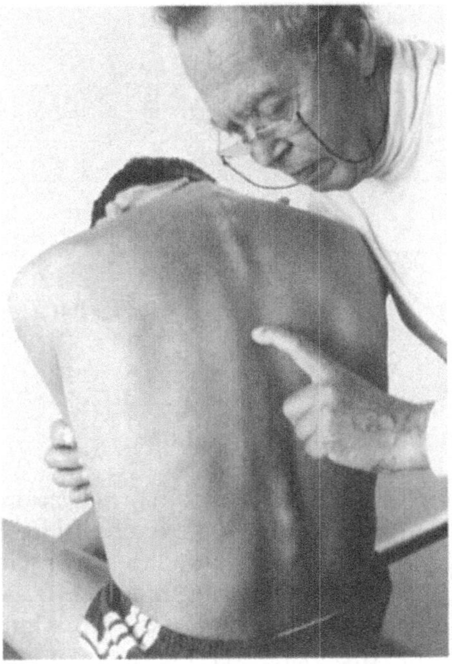

Fig. 157

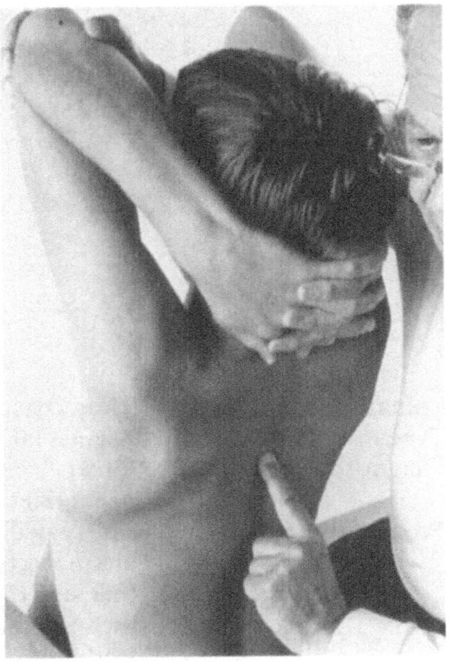

Fig. 158

Spinal Area: Thoracic spine
Type of Examination: Segmental motion testing for sidebending
Diagnostic Usefulness: Great: USA, SWE, SWI, FRG, F
Procedure: American variation: the examiner stands at the side of the upright seated patient. The thumb and index finger are placed together forming a "V" over the interspinous region. With his other hand, the examiner introduces maximal passive sidebending of the head (Fig. 159) evaluating the mobility of the spinous processes in the contra-lateral direction (evaluating the coupled motion of rotation and sidebending). Czechoslovakian variation: the examiner palpates the spinous process at the concave side with his thumb (Fig. 160).

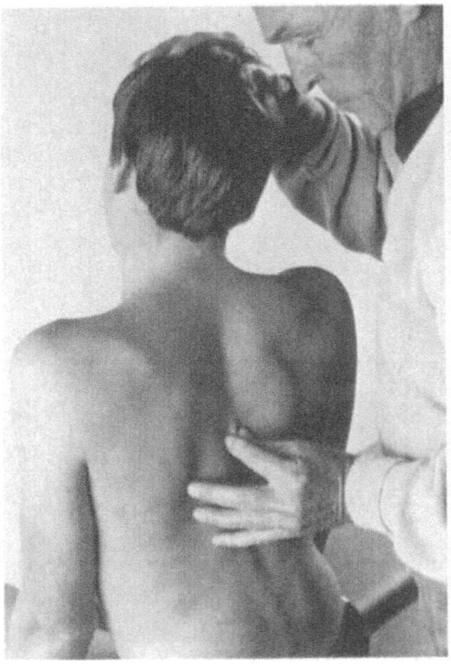

Fig. 159

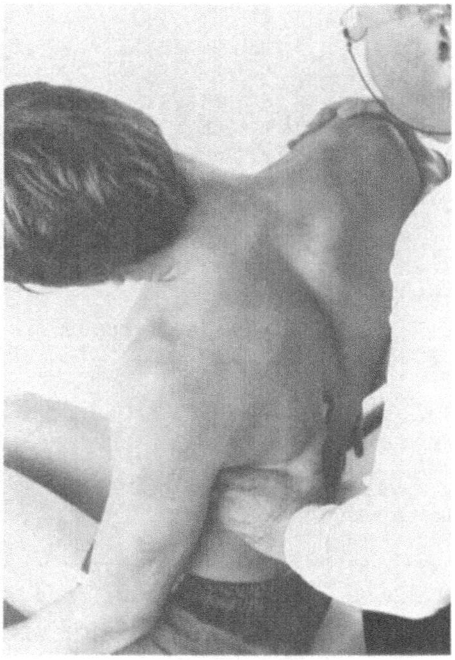

Fig. 160

Spinal Area: Thoracic spine
Type of Examination: Segmental motion testing for rotation
Diagnostic Usefulness: Great: USA, SWE, CZE
Moderate: FRG and F only for pain provocation
Procedure: The seated patient is in a slightly flexed position. First, the spinous processes are inspected, as the patient is asked to actively rotate his upper body to either side (Fig. 161). Two adjoining spinous processes are then palpated with the index and middle fingers, and passive rotation to the left and right are introduced. During this maneuver, the range of motion of individual spinous processes is evaluated (USA variation: Fig. 162; Czechoslovakian variation: Figs. 163, 164).

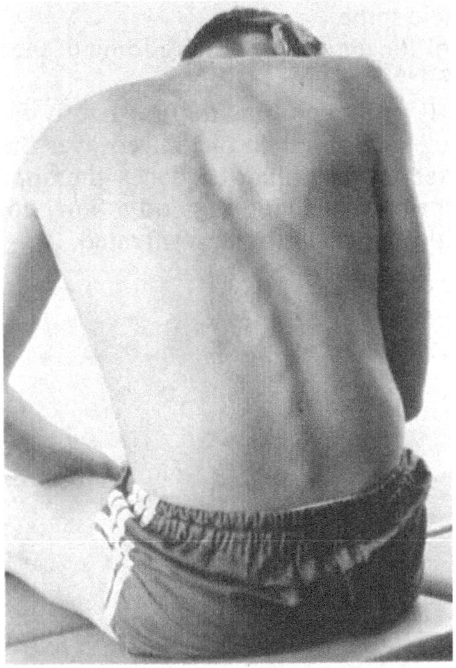

Fig. 161

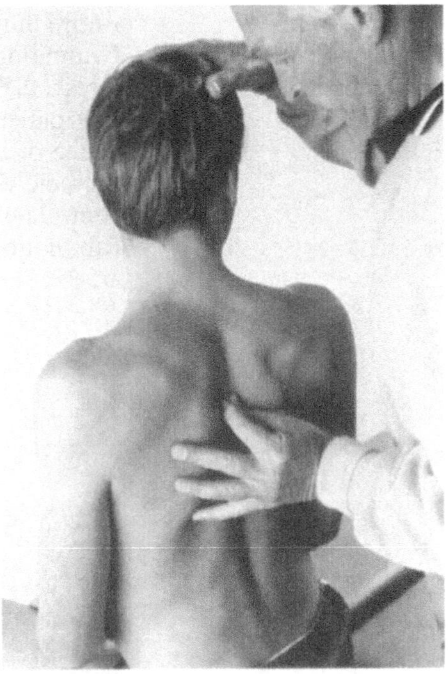

Fig. 162

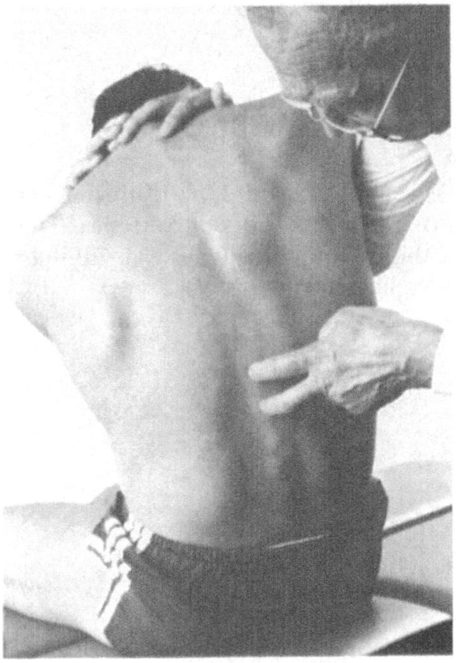

Fig. 163

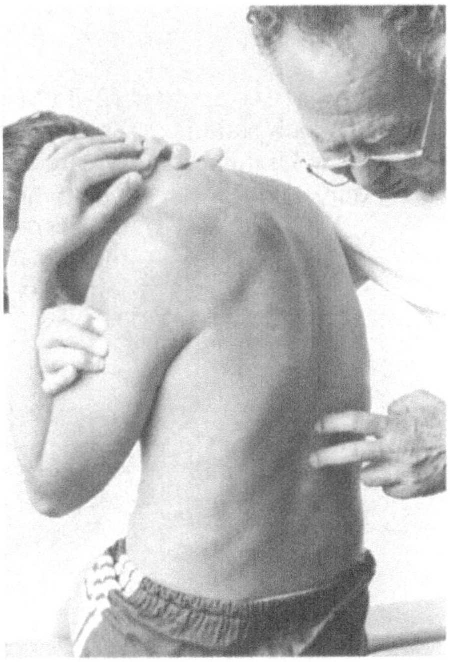

Fig. 164

Spinal Area: Entire thoracic spine
Type of Examination: Evaluation of the antero-posterior gliding of the costo-transverse joints
Diagnostic Usefulness: Great: SWE
Procedure: The patient is prone with his thorax slightly flexed. The hypothenar eminence of the examining hand is placed over the transverse process of one thoracic vertebrae. The ulnar border of the opposite hand is placed on the contralateral rib establishing as good a bony contact as possible (Fig. 165). Rib motion during respiration is evaluated.

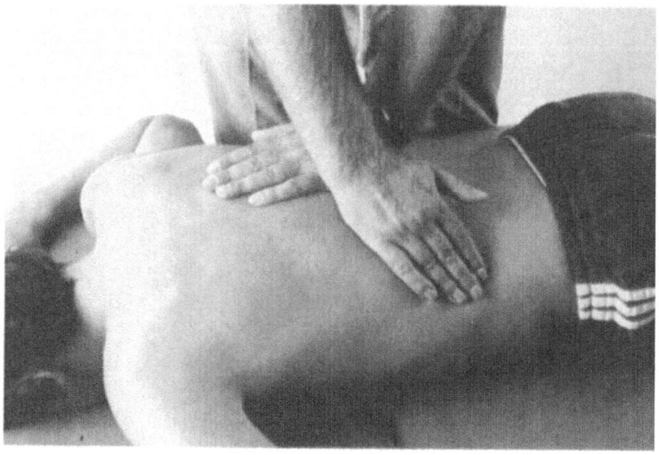

Fig. 165

Spinal Area: T2–T12
Type of Examination: Springing test of the tranverse process
Diagnostic Usefulness: Great: USA
Procedure: The patient is seated upright. One thumb is accurately positioned over the transverse process of one thoracic vertebra. The other thumb is placed over the palpating thumb and introduces a springing motion (Fig. 166). Segmental joint play is evaluated.

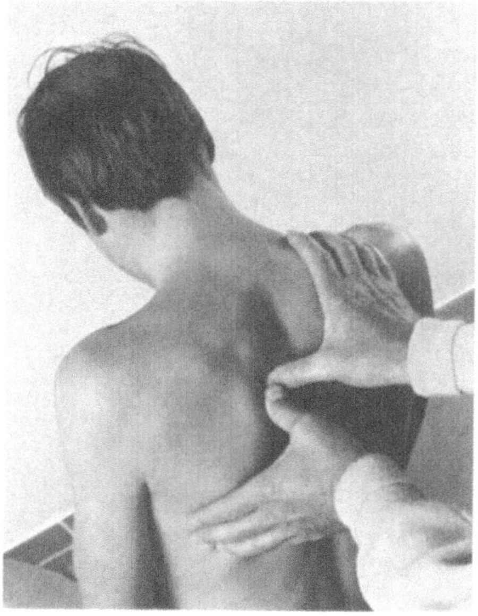

Fig. 166

Spinal Area: Thoracic spine
Type of Examination: Rib motion testing during inhalation and exhalation
Diagnostic Usefulness: Moderate: SWI
Procedure: The patient is prone, with his thorax slightly flexed. Starting from above (cephilad), the examiner's palm establishes good bony contact with the individual ribs (Fig. 167). The symmetry of rib motion is compared during inhalation and exhalation.

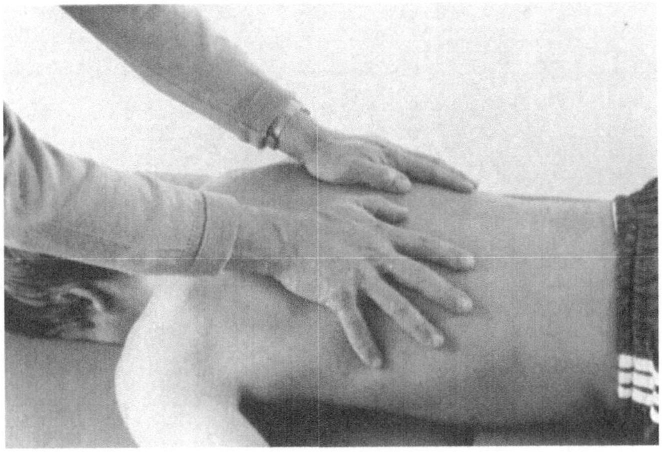

Fig. 167

Spinal Area: Ribs and thorax
Type of Examination: Evaluation of rib motion during respiration
Diagnosis Usefulness: Great: F
Procedure: The patient, is sitting upright, and leans with one axilla over the examiner's thigh who stands behind the patient with one leg at the patient's side. Starting superiorly the examiner palpates the lateral third of the individual ribs with his thumbs and tests the mobility of the individual ribs during inhalation and exhalation (Fig. 168). Then, the examiner places the palpating index fingers (starting inferiorly) again on the lateral third of the individual ribs (Fig. 169) and once more evaluates mobility during inhalation and exhalation. If pain appears during the course of the examination it provides an important finding to the examiner in the diagnostic workup.

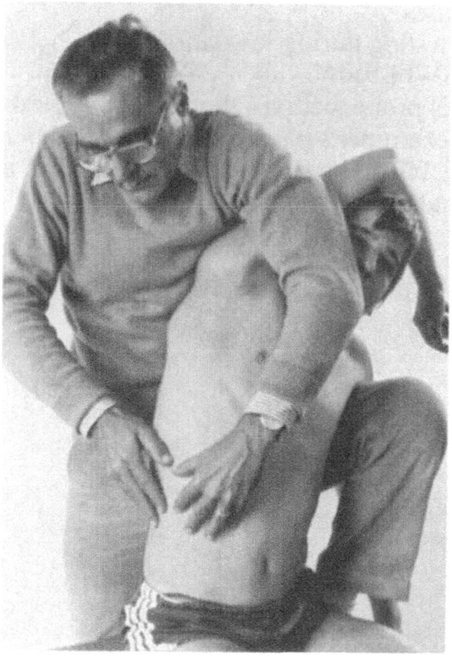

Fig. 168

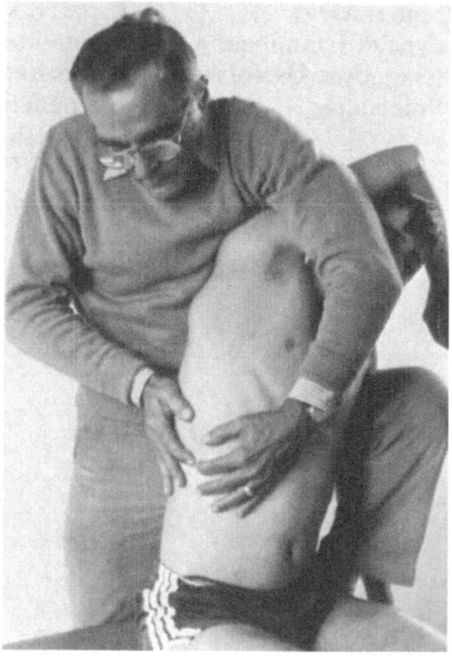

Fig. 169

Spinal Area: Ribs and thorax
Type of Examination: Rib motion testing with simultaneous passive rotation of the upper arm
Diagnosis Usefulness: Great: SWE
Procedure: The fingers of the palpating hand are placed intercostally and parasternally over the individual intercostal spaces of the seated patient. The patient is instructed to elevate and abduct his upper arm at the shoulder, as the range of motion of the individual ribs is evaluated (Fig. 170). The arm is then passively elevated 90°, the elbow is flexed 90°, and rotated both internally and externally. During this procedure, the anterior-posterior motion of the individual ribs is evaluated (Fig. 171).

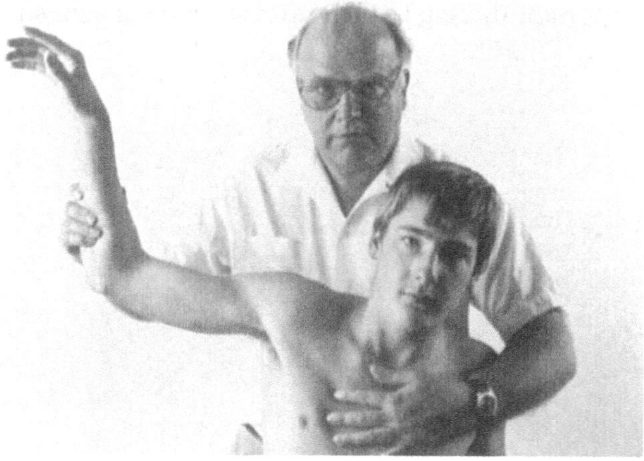

Fig. 170

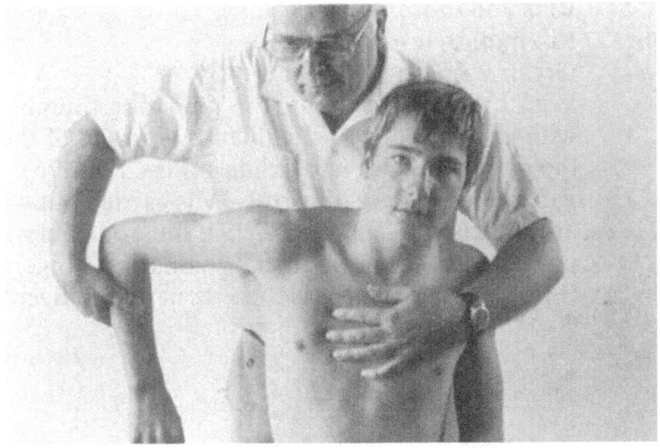

Fig. 171

Spinal Area: Ribs and thorax
Type of Examination: Rib motion during inhalation and exhalation
Diagnostic Usefulness: Great: USA
Procedure: The patient is sitting upright. The examiner stands behind the patient and places both hands over the lateral third of the anterior aspect of the individual ribs to allow a comparison of individual rib motion (Fig. 172). The examiner then palpates the posterior aspect of the upper ribs (Fig. 173) and again evaluates the range of motion of the individual ribs while the patient inhales and exhales.

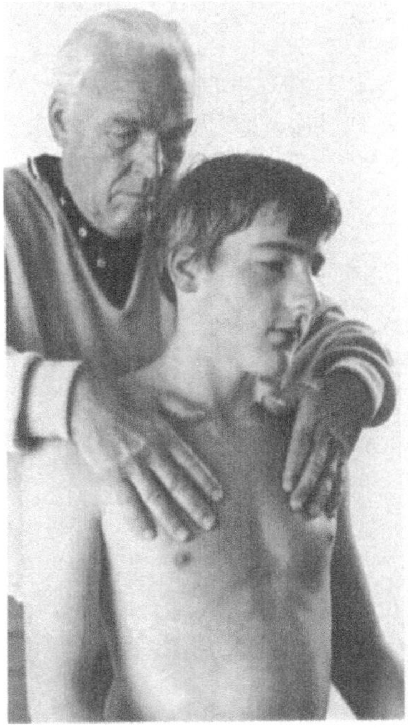

Fig. 172

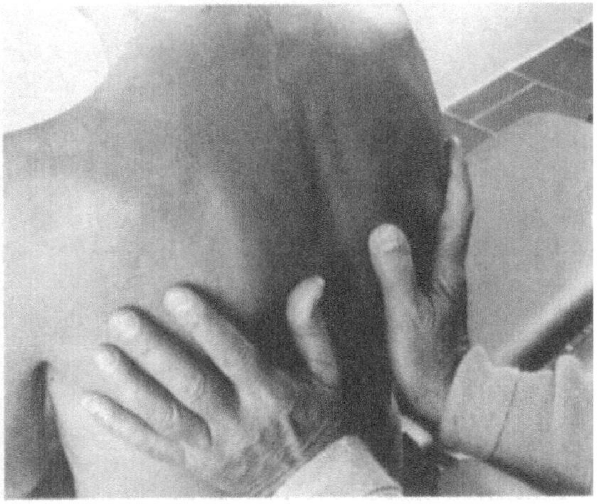

Fig. 173

Spinal Area: Ribs and thorax
Type of Examination: Rib motion testing
Diagnostic Usefulness: Great: CZE
Procedure: With the patient supine, the palpating thumbs are placed in close contact with one pair of ribs. Evaluation is made of the symmetry of rib motion as the patient inhales and exhales (Figs. 174, 175).
Rib motion testing for ribs I–IV is carried out with the patient seated and the arm maximally elevated. While the arm is elevated and passively extended posteriorly, the examiner's palpating fingers resist upper rib motion (Fig. 176). The patient is then requested to deeply inhale and exhale.

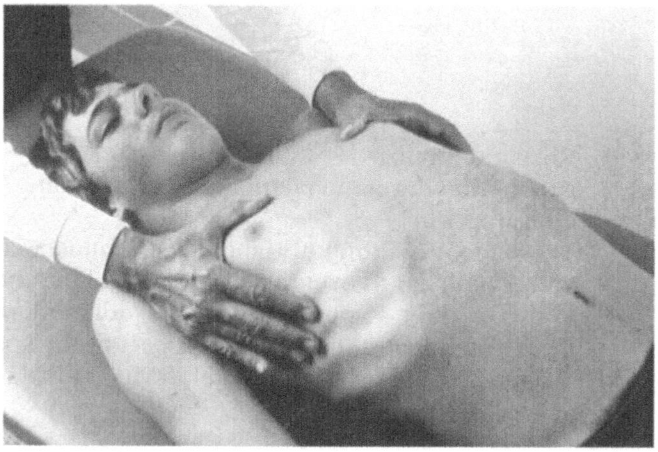

Fig. 174

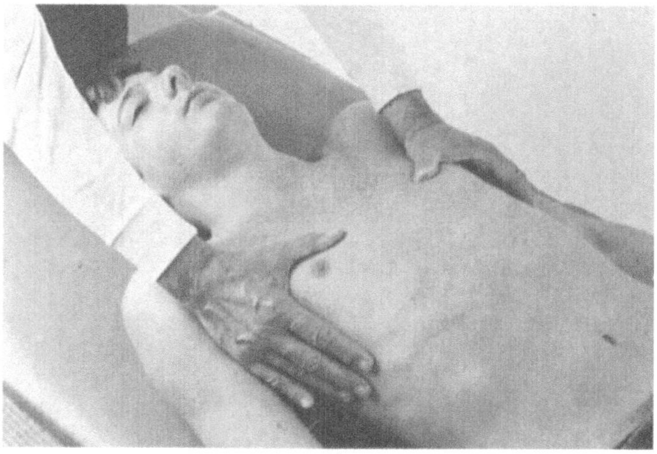

Fig. 175

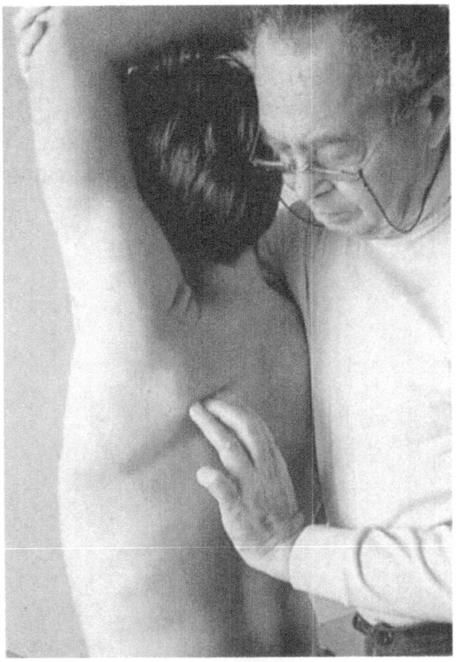

Fig. 176

Spinal Area: Ribs
Type of Examination: Rib motion testing, sitting
Diagnostic Usefulness: Moderate: FRG
Procedure: The examiner stands behind the seated patient. The patient drapes one arm over the examiner's thigh while the contralateral arm is elevated. The examiner's palpating fingers are placed over the lateral third of the individual ribs evaluating the intercostal spaces during maximal inhalation and exhalation (Fig. 177).

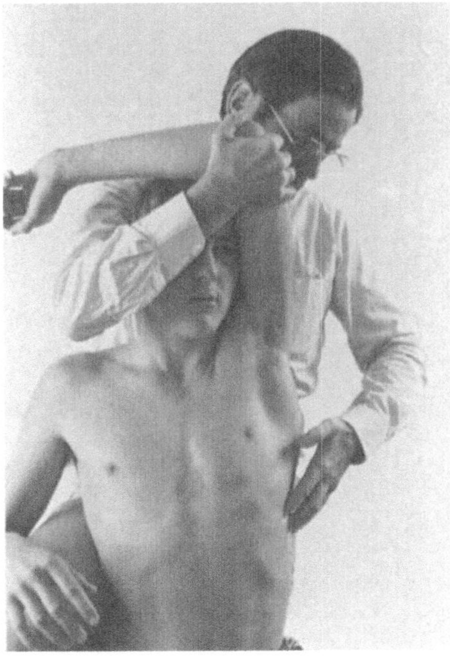

Fig. 177

Spinal Area: Ribs
Type of Examination: Rib motion testing in the costo-transverse joints
Diagnostic Usefulness: Great: FRG, SWE, SWI, USA
Procedure: The patient is prone with his thoracic spine slightly flexed. Starting superiorly, the fingertips are placed over the costal angle (Fig. 178). The individual inter-costal spaces and changes with respiration are evaluated.

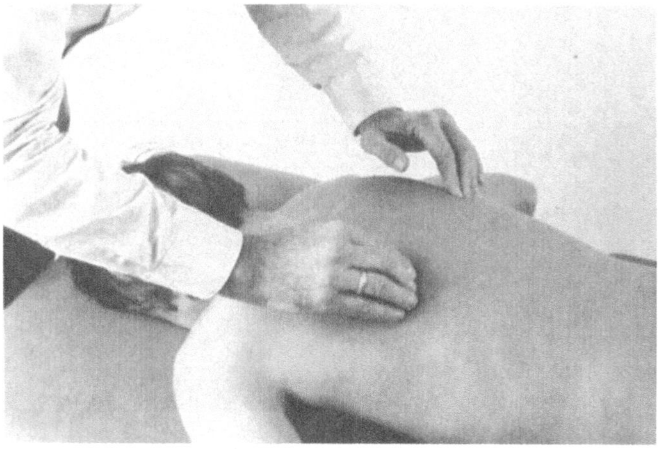

Fig. 178

Spinal Area: Ribs, anterior and lateral portions
Type of Examination: Rib motion testing (ribs I–IV anterior, ribs V–X lateral)
Diagnostic Usefulness: Great: FRG, SWE, CZE
Procedure: The patient is supine. The examiner palpates the lateral and sternal third of the ribs (Fig. 179). Evaluation is made of the intercostal spaces during inhalation and exhalation to assess any motion restrictions.

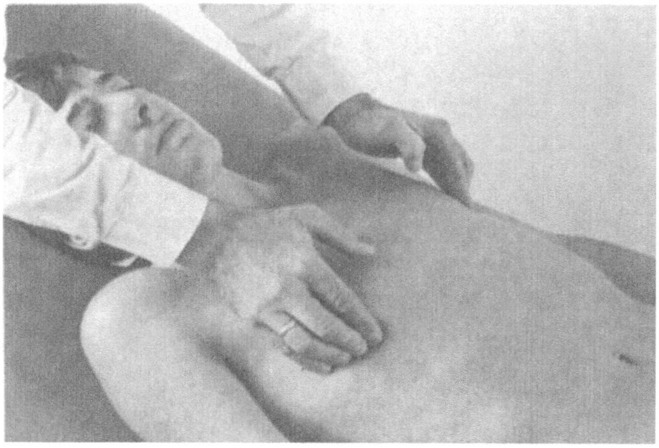

Fig. 179

5.2.4 Neuromuscular Examination

Spinal Area: Thoracic inlet

Type of Examination: Length testing of the pectoralis major muscle

Diagnostic Usefulness: Great: CZE, SWE, SWI, DEN
Moderate: F, USA

Procedure: The patient is supine. While the patient's thorax is stabilized with one of the examiner's forearms, the patient's arm is supinated and moved superiorly with the examiner's other hand (Fig. 180) following the direction of the pectoralis major muscle fibers (the American school only evaluates muscular tension without passive elevation of the arm). During this procedure, the index and middle fingers palpate the mid portion of the pectoralis major muscle evaluating the resistence or manifestation of tenderness (Fig. 181).

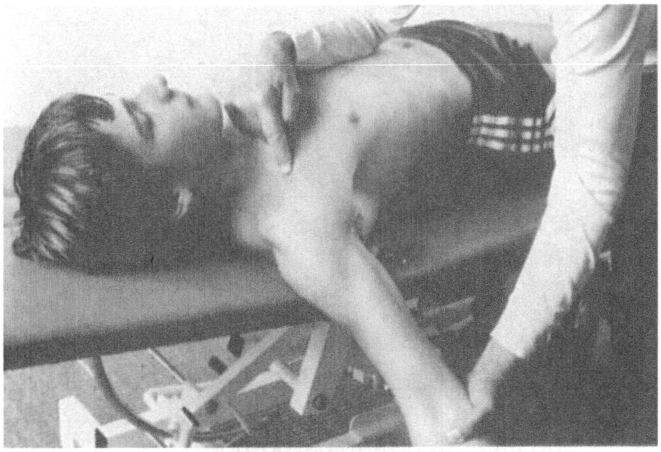

Fig. 180

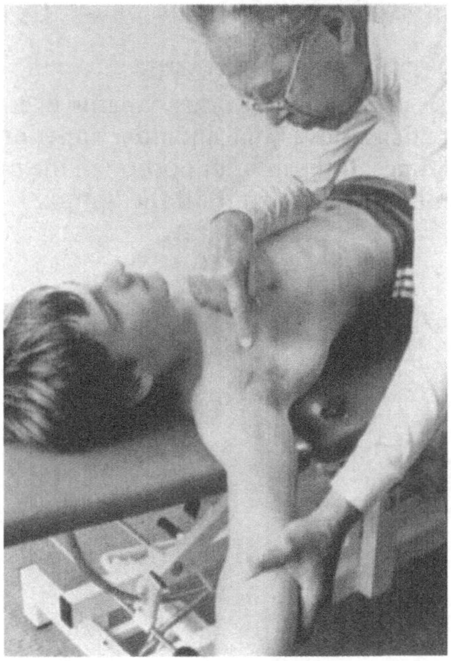

Fig. 181

Spinal Area: Upper and mid thoracic spine

Type of Examination: Testing for muscle strength of the interscapular muscles and the serratus anterior muscle

Diagnostic Usefulness: Great: SWI, CZE, FRG, USA, SWE

Procedure: The patient rests on his elbows and knees with the hands rotated medially and the weight distributed over the arms. The scapulae are abducted. The patient remains in this position. If one finds that the scapula is more posterior on one side, the interscapular muscles are weakened (including rhomboid minor and major muscles, the horizontal and ascending portions of the trapezius muscle and the anterior serratus muscle) (Fig. 182).

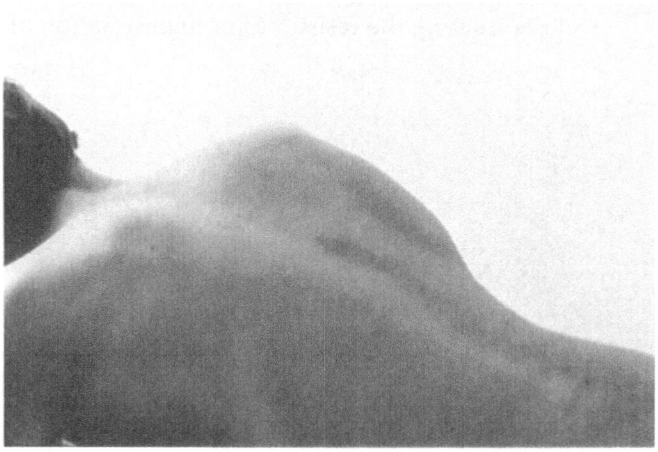

Fig. 182

Spinal Area: Mid and lower thoracic portion

Type of Examination: Testing for strength of the trapezius muscle (horizontal and ascending portions)

Diagnostic Usefulness: Great: SWI, CZE, FRG, USA, SWE

Procedure: The patient is prone with his arms hanging over the side of the examination table. The patient moves one shoulder superiorly and inferiorly (Figs. 183, 184) several times. If the inferior portion of the trapezius muscle is weakened the shoulder blade tends to lift off the thorax.

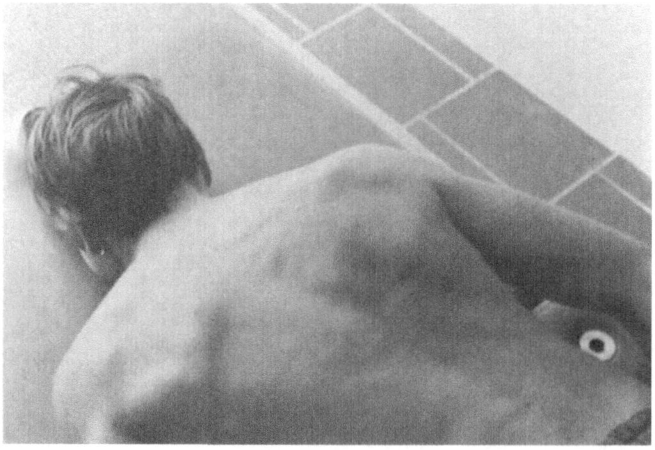

Fig. 183

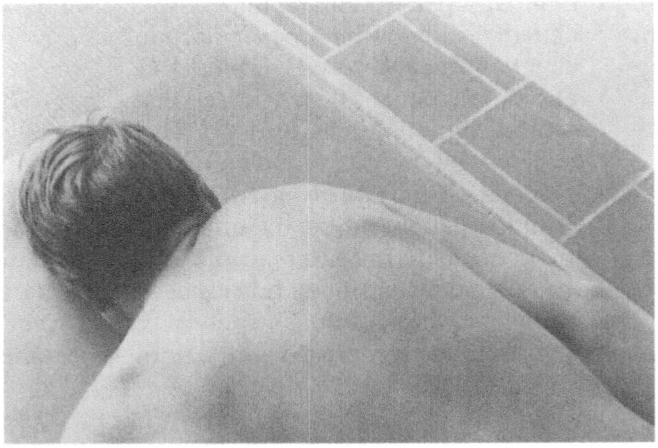

Fig. 184

Spinal Area:	Thoraco-lumbar junction
Type of Examination:	Length testing of the quadratus lumborum muscle
Diagnostic Usefulness:	Great: CZE, FRG, SWI, USA, SWE
Procedure:	Screening test: the patient is standing and actively sidebends to one side maximally. A general impression of the range of motion is obtained (Fig. 185). For a more specific examination, the patient starts in the sidelying position and then pushes himself up by his elbow which is next to the table until the superior-iliac crest (the crest farthest from the table's surface) moves inferiorly (Fig. 186). This test is repeated on the other side, and asymmetry of motion is evaluated.

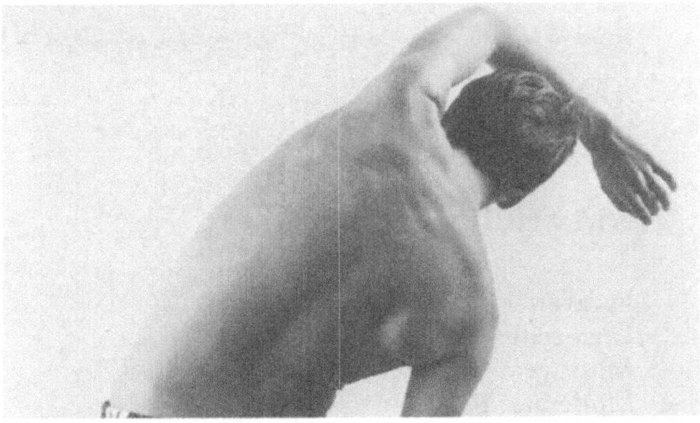

Fig. 185

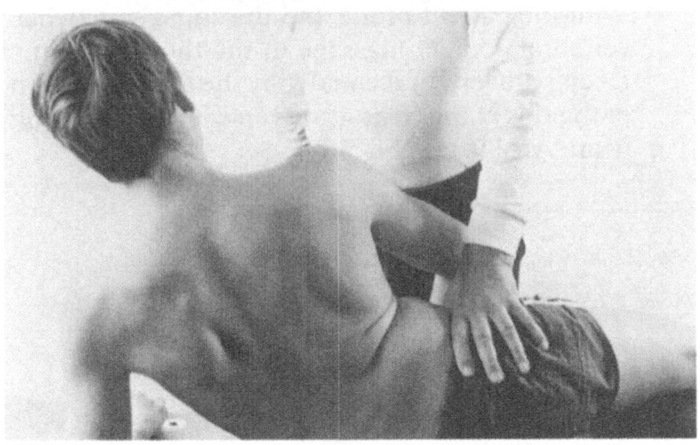

Fig. 186

Spinal Area: Lumbar – pelvis – hip region
Type of Examination: Length testing of the psoas major muscle
Diagnostic Usefulness: Great: CZE, SWI, SWE, USA, FRG
Procedure: The supine patient flexes the leg that is not to be tested on the thorax, thus neutralizing the lumbarlordosis. The leg that is to be examined is extended horizontally on the examination table while the foreleg, being flexed 90°, is dropped off the table (Fig. 187).
With the patient prone, the lumbarlordosis is neutralized (a small pillow or the patient's hands are placed under the abdomen): evaluation is made of the range of extension of one leg at a time while the buttocks on the opposite side is stabilized.
Remarks: This is not to be confused with painful syndromes of L3–L4 seen with the reserved Lasegue test.

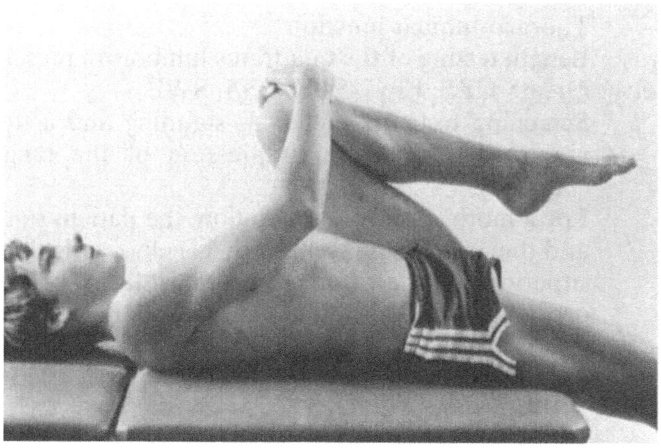

Fig. 187

5.3 Therapy

5.3.1 Soft Tissue Treatment

Type of Treatment: Paravertebral contact massage
Goal: Unspecific muscle relaxation
Technique: Massage
Therapeutic Usefulness: Moderate: F
Procedure: With the patient prone and the spine somewhat flexed, one performs paravertebral contact massage to the thoracic spine including rib mobilization. Deep paravertebral contact by the thenar eminence leads to the mobilization of the ribs at the costo-transverse joint by moving from superiorly to inferiorly and vice versa (Fig. 188).

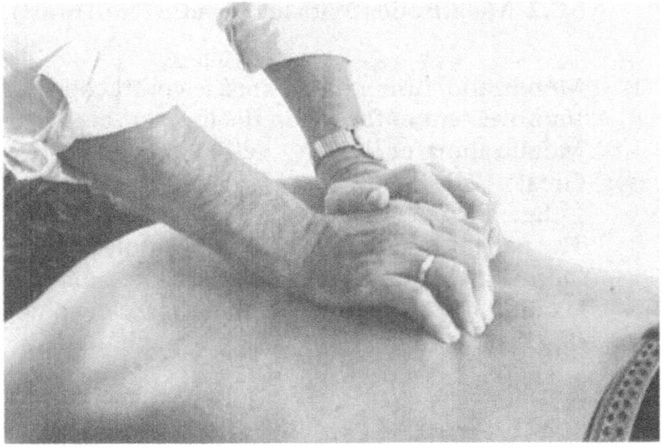

Fig. 188

Type of Treatment:	Deep paravertebral massage
Goal:	To decrease muscle tension in the erector-spine system
Technique:	"Deep pressure inhibition"
Therapeutic Usefulness:	Great: USA
	Moderate: FRG, SWE
Procedure:	The patient lies on one side. The tight paravertebral muscles are palpated with the fingertips and lateral stretch is applied and then released to effect a decrease in muscle tone (Fig. 189). The procedure is repeated until adequate relaxation is effected.

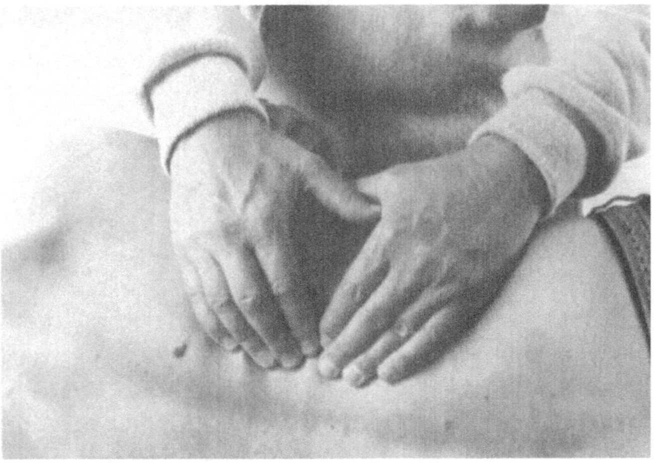

Fig. 189

5.3.2 Mobilization Without Impulse (No Thrust)

Type of Treatment: Mobilization using direct muscle contraction
Goal: Improvement of flexion in the thoracic area
Technique: Mobilization for flexion – self mobilization
Therapeutic Usefulness: Great: CZE
Little: FRG
Procedure: The patient is in the knee-chest position with both arms stretched inferiorly. During inspiration, flexion of the thoracic spine is emphasized (Fig. 190), relaxation or extension of the thoracic spine occurs during exhalation (Fig. 191).

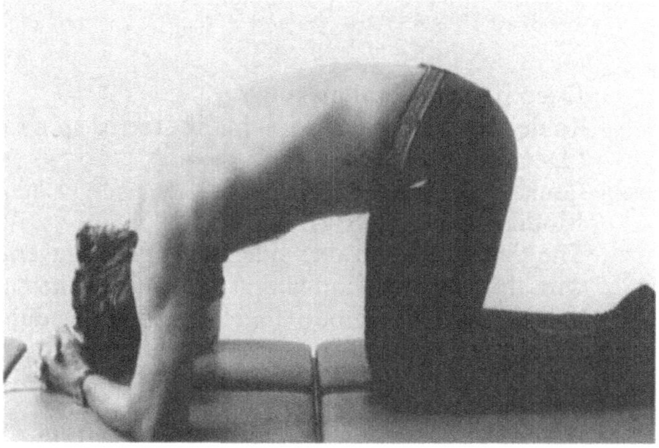

Fig. 190

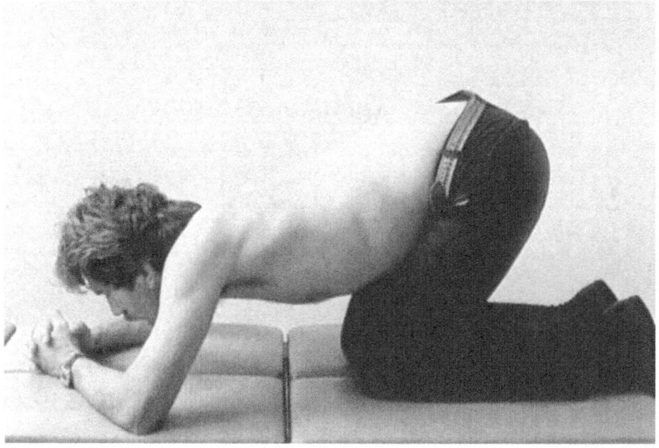

Fig. 191

Type of Treatment: Mobilization using direct muscle contraction
Goal: Improvement of extension motion in the thoracic spine
Technique: Extension mobilization – self mobilization
Therapeutic Usefulness: Great: SWE, CZE, FRG
Procedure: The patient rests his thoracic spine against the back of a chair. The height of the chair support is determined by the level of the spinal segment to be mobilized. Both arms are abducted approximately 70°.
Simultaneous inhalation and supination cause the thoracic spine to extend. The back support of the chair acts as a stabilizing counterforce. During exhalation, pronation and internal rotation of the arms is carried out as the thoracic spine relaxes.

Type of Treatment: Mobilization using direct muscle contraction
Goal: Improvement extension in the thoracic spine
Technique: Extension mobilization – self mobilization
Therapeutic Usefulness: Great: CZE
Little: FRG
None: USA
Procedure: The patient is seated and his arms are abducted 70°. Inhalation and supination with external rotation of both arms all increase extension of the thoracic spine. During exhalation and internal rotation with pronation of the arms, the erector spinae muscles in the thoracic region relax. The mid thoracic spine is mobilized in this maneuver (Fig. 192).

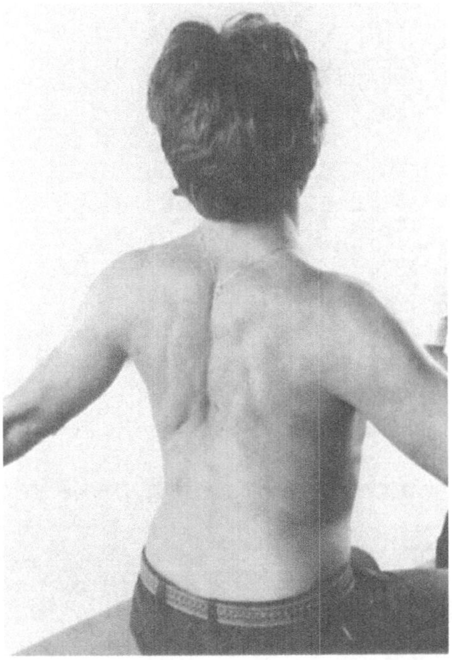

Fig. 192

Type of Treatment:	Mobilization without impulse
Goal:	Improvement of extension
Technique:	Extension mobilization
Therapeutic Usefulness:	Great: F, FRG Moderate: USA, SWE Little: SWI, CZE
Procedure:	The patient is seated with his arms crossed over his forehead. Using both hands, the operator's fingers make contact at either one (i.e., T9, Fig. 193) or at several transverse processes (Fig. 194). The operator performs traction and anterior pressure simultaneously with both hands.
Remarks:	Depending on the final position of the spine, the operator can vary this method and introduce rotation mobilization or sidebending mobilization. Post-isometric relaxation can be utilized with this type of mobilization if timed with the exhalation phase (Figs. 195, 196).

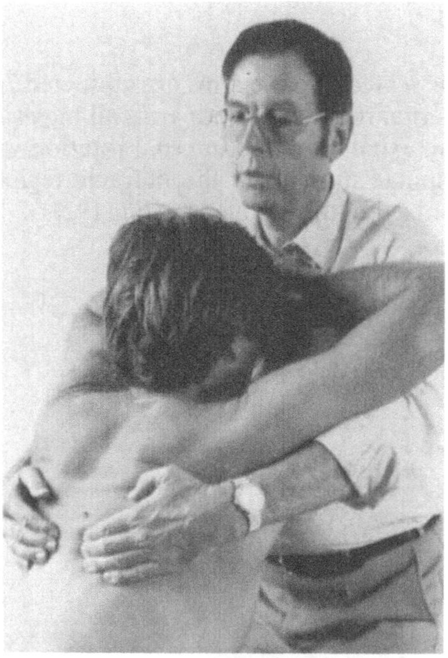

Fig. 193

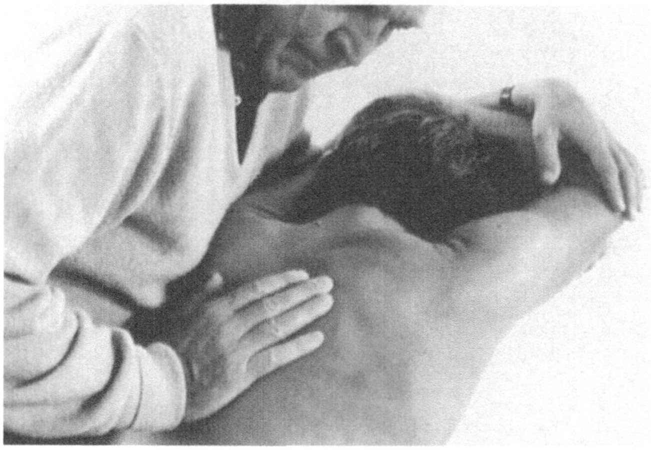

Fig. 194

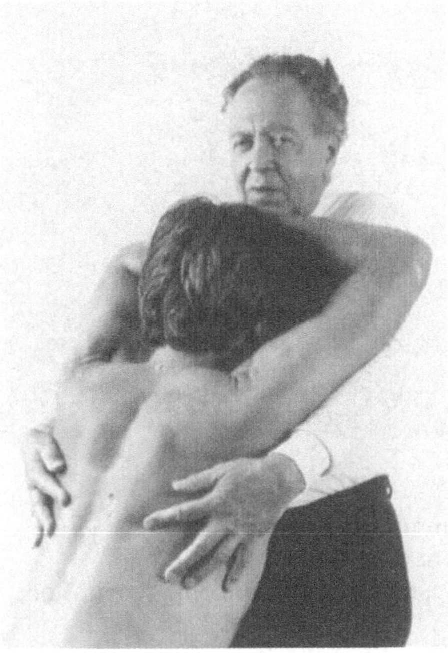

Fig. 195

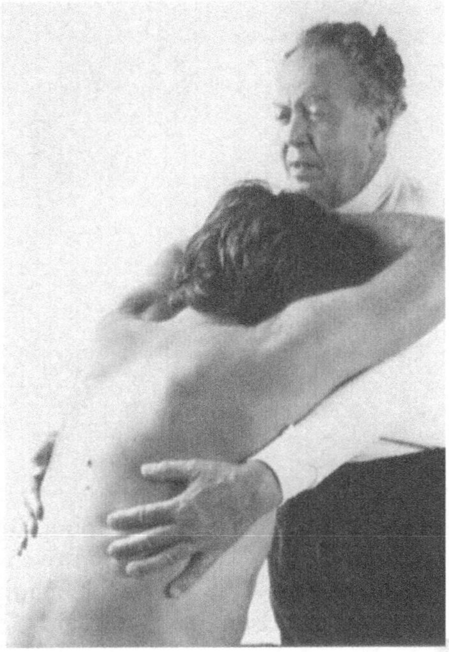

Fig. 196

Type of Treatment:	Extension mobilization utilizing respiratory effort
Goal:	Improvement of extension in the thoracic spine
Technique:	Extension mobilization with application of respiration movement
Therapeutic Usefulness:	Great: CZE None: FRG, F, SWI
Procedure:	The patient is in the side-lying position. Inhalation is carried out until the segment to be stabilized is reached (Fig. 197). This is followed by maximal exhalation and passive extension mobilization (Fig. 198).

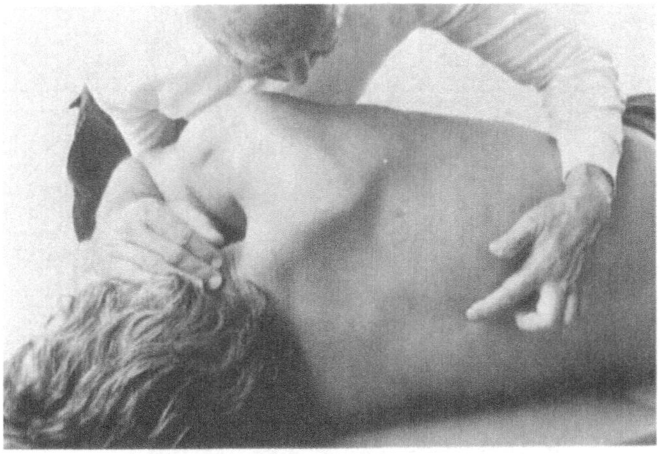

Fig. 197

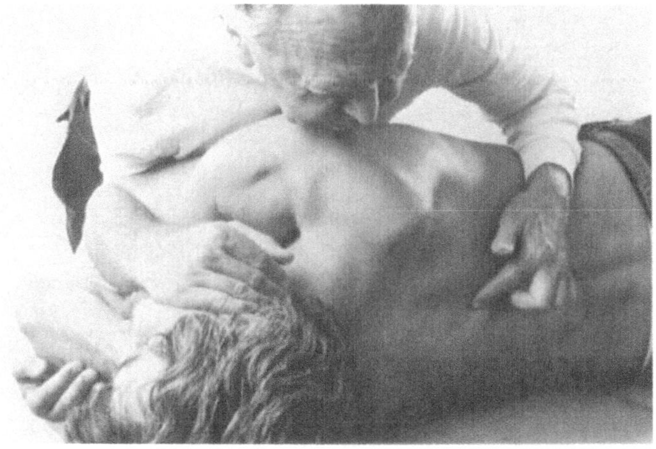

Fig. 198

Type of Treatment:	Mobilization utilizing respiration
Goal:	Improvement of thoracic sidebending
Technique:	Sidebending, mobilization utilizing respiration
Therapeutic Usefulness:	Great: CZE None: FRG, SWE, SWI, F
Procedure:	The operator stabilizes the patient's thorax laterally with his whole hand while he fixes the spinous process with the thumb. The other hand introduces sidebending in the patient's trunk (Fig. 199). For a neutral segment, the procedure is as follows: the patient moves superiorly and breathes only shallowly. During exhalation mobilization and relaxation occur. With a non-neutral segment, the patient first exhales, thereby increasing resistance. It is during the inspiratory motion that relaxation and mobilization occur.

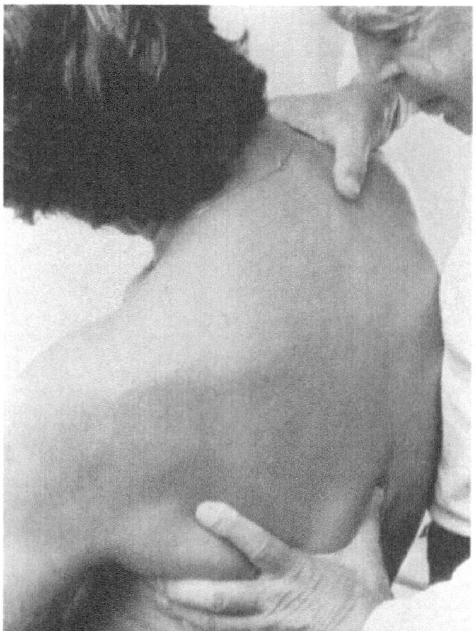

Fig. 199

Type of Treatment: Mobilization without impulse
Goal: General mobilization to improve rotation in the thoracic spine
Technique: Rotation mobilization
Therapeutic Usefulness: Great: USA, F
Moderate: SWE, SWI
Little: CZE
None: FRG
Procedure: The patient is seated. The operator places one palm over the patient's paravertebral musculature in the thoracic region while the other hand holds the shoulder girdle (Fig. 200).
Force is applied to the thorax in an anterolateral direction, and the shoulder is simultaneously rotated to enhance overall thorax rotation.

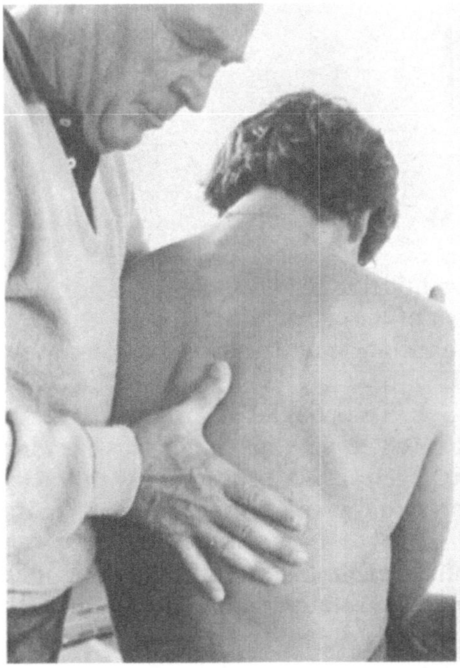

Fig. 200

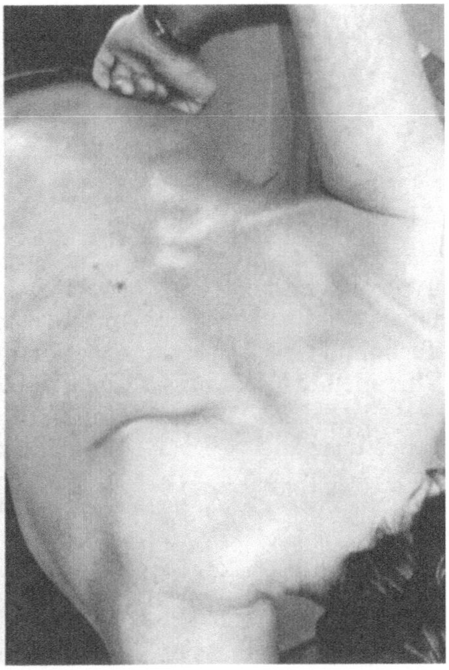

Fig. 201

Type of Treatment: Mobilization utilizing direct muscle contraction
Goal: Improvement of thoracic rotation (in this example, to the left side)
Technique: Rotation mobilization – self mobilization
Therapeutic Usefulness: Great: CZE, FRG
Little: SWE
None: USA, F
Procedure: In this example, the patient is in the knee-chest position and his left arm is abducted in the shoulder and flexed at the elbow.
Forced rotation is achieved by having the patient's head and neck turn to the left. The shoulder girdle is also rotatated (Fig. 201).

Type of Treatment: Mobilization without impulse
Goal: Improvement of thoracic rotation
Technique: Rotation mobilization

Therapeutic Usefulness: Great: USA, SWE
Moderate: FRG
Little: SWI, CZE

Procedure: In this example, the operator's right thumb makes bony contact with the transverse process of T8. The other hand (left) is used to increase pressure on the vertebra.
Mobilization in a lateral and anterior direction (Fig. 202).

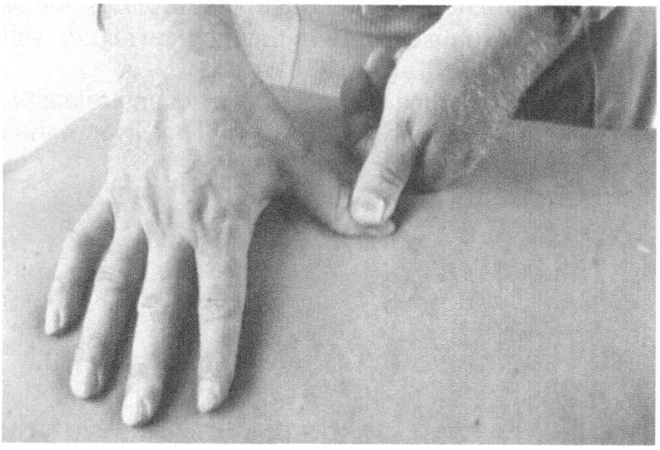

Fig. 202

Type of Treatment: Mobilization utilizing respiration
Goal: Improvement of thorax rotation
Technique: Rotation mobilization utilizing respiration
Therapeutic Usefulness Great: CZE
None: FRG, F, SWE, SWI

Procedure: The patient is seated with his hands clasp behind his neck. Rotation to one side (i.e., to the left) is introduced in the thoracic and lumbar spine. The operator's right thumb presses on the patient's thoracic vertebra (T9' for example).
After an initial deep inhalation motion, the operator's left hand introduces motion to increase rotation while the patient exhales (Fig. 203).

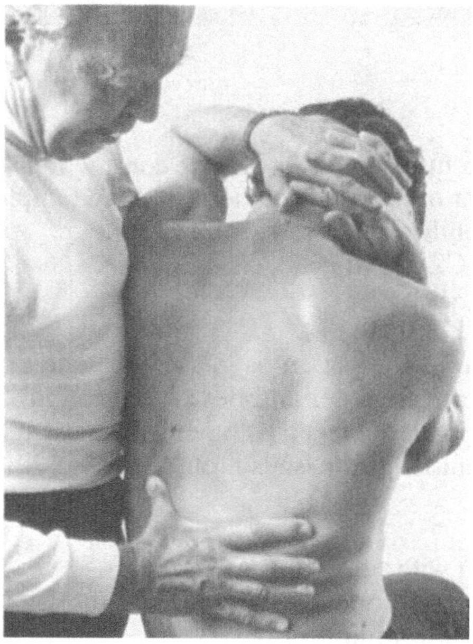

Fig. 203

Type of Treatment: Mobilization utilizing direct muscle contraction (psoas muscle)
Goal: Improvement of movement of thoraco-lumbar junction motion
Technique: Rotation mobilization – self mobilization
Therapeutic Usefulness: Great: SWE, CZE
Moderate: FRG
Procedure: In this example, the vertebral column of the supine patient is rotated to the left. The left hip is flexed and monitored at the knee joint with the operator's right hand. The psoas major muscle is activated by having the patient contract the upper thigh against his knee thereby improving restricted rotation at the thoraco-lumbar segments (Fig. 204).

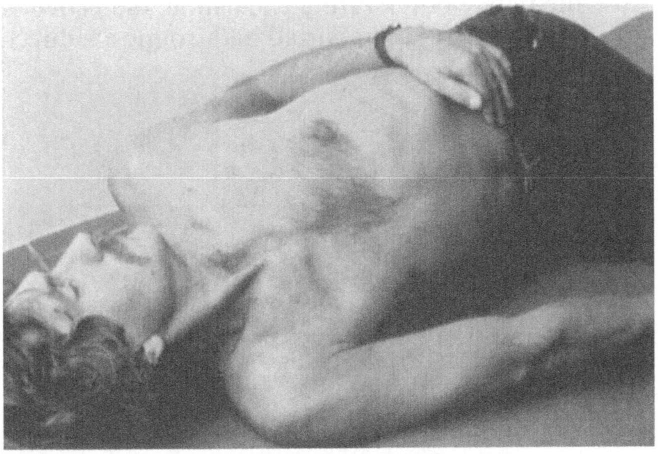

Fig. 204

Type of Treatment: Rib mobilization utilizing muscle contraction
Goal: Improvement of rib mobility (ribs V–X)
Technique: Rib mobilization
Therapeutic Usefulness: Great: FRG
Procedure: The patient is prone. In this example, the patient's right transverse process of T10 is stabilized with the operator's left hand. The pisiform bone of the operator's right hand makes contact with the patient's left tenth rib. The tenth rib on the left side is isometrically held in place during inhalation (Fig. 205). During exhalation, mobilization is effected over the costal angle in an anterior direction.

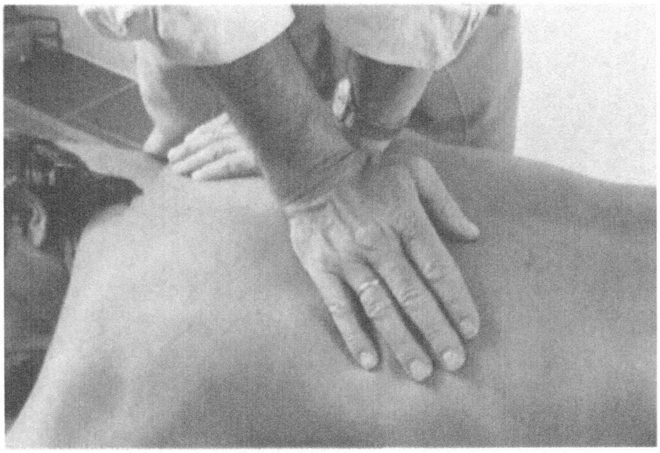

Fig. 205

Type of Treatment: Rib mobilization
Goal: Improvement of rib mobility
Technique: Rib mobilization utilizing respiration
Therapeutic Usefulness: Great: SWE, FRG
Moderate: SWI, CZE
Little: F

Procedure: The patient is in the lateral recumbant position. In this example, the patient's right arm is elevated maximally. The operator places his right hand over the patient's elbow. The restricted rib is held in place with the operator's index finger (Fig. 206).

During the inhalation movement, an isometric counterforce is established at the right elbow. During exhalation, the patient's right arm is elevated some more. The rib is mobilized in the opposite direction.

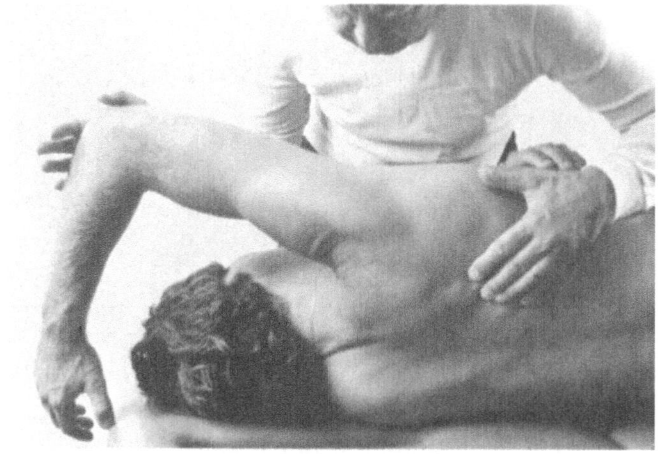

Fig. 206

Type of Treatment: Mobilization without impulse
Goal: Improvement of rib mobility
Technique: Rib mobilization during exhalation
Therapeutic Usefulness: Moderate: USA
None: SWI, FRG, F, SWE

Procedure: While prone, flexion is introduced in the patient's spine. The operator's thumb is placed over the costal angle of, i.e., the eighth rib. The hands rest broadly over the ribs on both sides (Fig. 207).

During exhalation an infero-anteriorly directed mobilizing force is introduced through both hands.

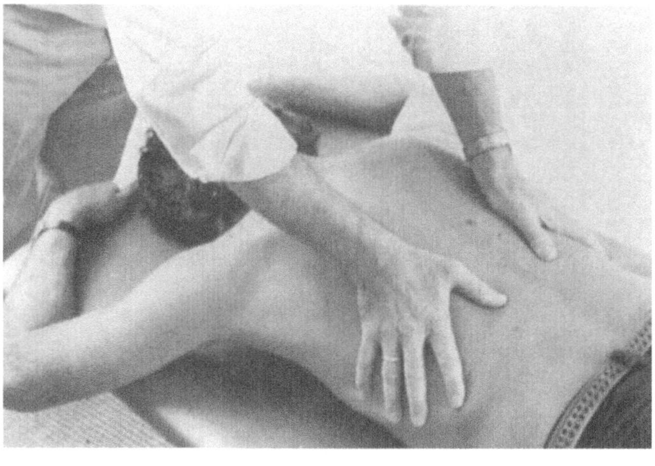

Fig. 207

Type of Treatment: Mobilization utilizing muscle energy techniques (MET) for the pectoralis minor and serratus anterior muscles

Goal: Improvement of rib motion during exhalation

Technique: Rib mobilization (Ribs II–X)

Therapeutic Usefulness:
Great: FRG, USA
Moderate: SWE, CZE
Little: F
None: SWI

Procedure: The patient is supine. In this example, the dorsum of the operator's hand stabilizes the costal angle of the restricted rib. The other hand rests broadly over the anterior thorax (Fig. 208). At the end of exhalation, mobilization is introduced at the costal angle in an inferior direction.

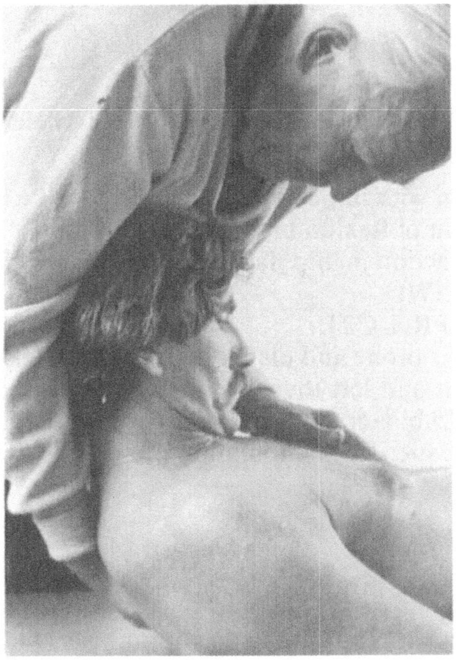

Fig. 208

Type of Treatment: Mobilization utilizing muscle contraction

Goal: Improvement of rib mobility during inhalation

Technique: Rib mobilization (Ribs III–IX)

Therapeutic Usefulness:
Great: FRG, USA
Moderate: SWE, CZE
Little: F
None: SWI

Procedure: In this example, the patient's right arm is abducted and flexed at the elbow. The right rib is localized dorsally by the operator's left hand. The patient's abducted arm is stabilized with the operator's right hand (Fig. 209).
The patient is instructed to inhale and exhale deeply. During inhalation the rib is mobilized by a downward force on the rib posteriorly to effect an elevation of the rib anteriorly.

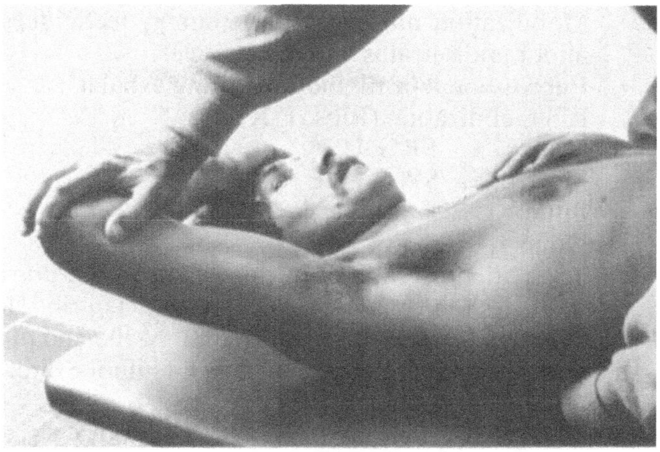

Fig. 209

5.3.3 Mobilization With Impulse (Thrust Techniques)

Type of Treatment: Mobilization with impulse
Goal: Improvement of flexion in the thoracic spine
Technique: Flexion – traction manipulation
Therapeutic Usefulness: Moderate: SWI
None: FRG, CZE
Procedure: The patient is prone and his thoracic spine is flexed. In this example, the operator's right and left thenar eminances make contract with the transverse process of T9 bilaterally (Fig. 210). The impulse is directed superiorly.
Remarks: This is not a specific manipulation procedure.

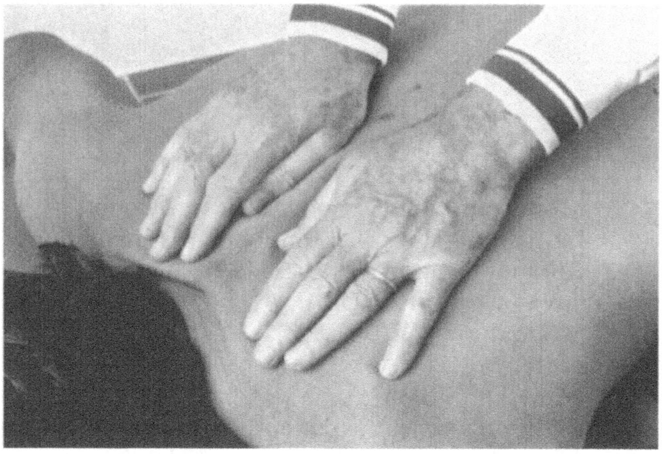

Fig. 210

Type of Treatment: Mobilization with impulse (thrust)
Goal: Improvement of extension in the thoracic spine
Technique: Extension manipulation
Therapeutic Usefulness: Great: FRG, SWE, CZE, SWI, FIN
Procedure: The patient is supine. Both the thenar eminence and the flexed middle finger of the operator are placed over the transverse processes bilaterally (Fig. 211). The thrusting force is directed posteriorly and is effected through the patient's crossed upper arms and shoulder girdle (Fig. 212).

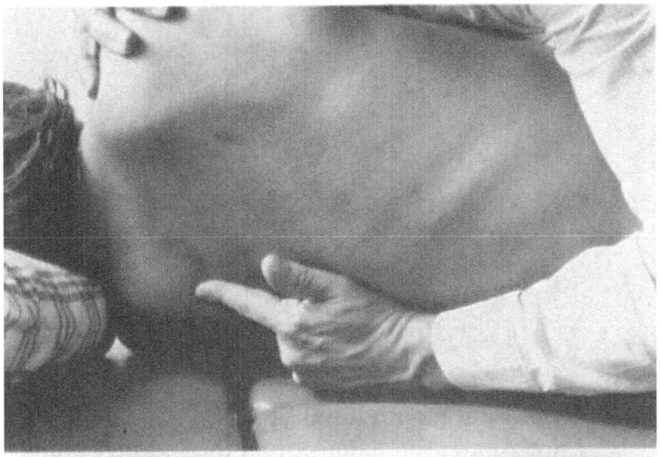

Fig. 211

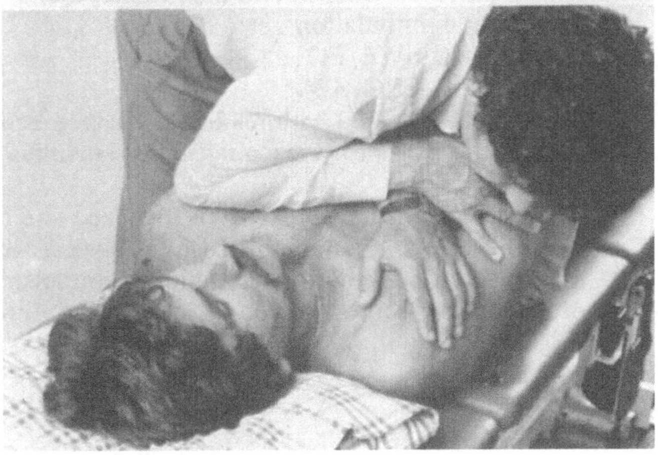

Fig. 212

Type of Treatment: Mobilization with impulse (thrust)
Goal: Improvement of extension in the thoracic spine
Technique: Extension manipulation
Therapeutic Usefulness: Great: USA, CZE, SWE, FIN
Moderate: SWI
None: FRG
Procedure: The patient is seated. A small towel or sandsack is placed at the interspinous interval. The operator's epigastric area is placed in contact with the towel. The patient is secured with the operator's hand clasping the patient's wrist with one hand while the other hand reaches under the opposite axilla to contact the patient's neck (Fig. 213).
The impulse is effected by the anterior movement of the operator's epigastric area with simultaneous upward traction through the operator's arms.

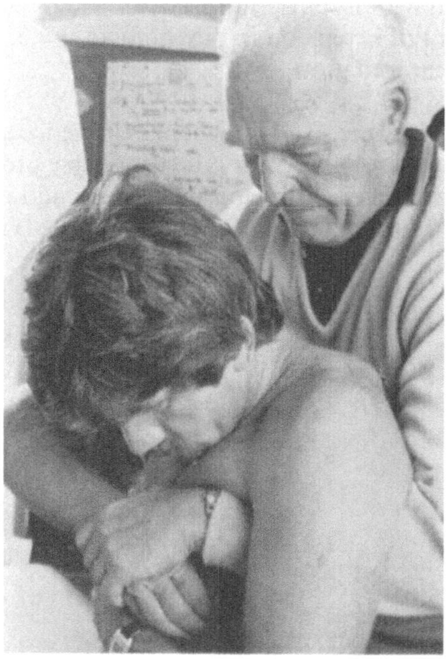

Fig. 213

Type of Treatment:	Mobilization with impulse
Goal:	Improvement of extension in the thoracic spine
Technique:	Extension manipulation
Therapeutic Usefulness:	Great: USA, SWE, FIN Little: CZE, FRG, SWI
Procedure:	The patient is seated with his hands clasped behind his neck. The operator secures the patient by reaching under his axilla to seize the patient's forearms. The spinal segment (i.e., T8–9) is localized and carried to its restrictive barrier. The operator's tibial tuberosity is placed over the spinous process (T9). The operator's knee provides a minimal impulse in an anterior direction. Simultaneously some traction is introduced through the operator's arms (Fig. 214).

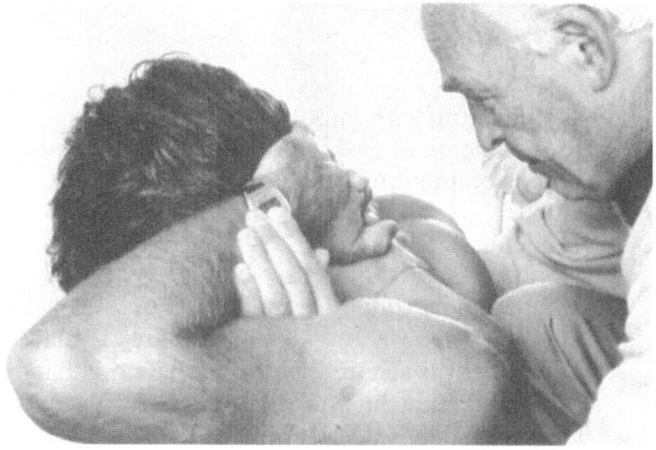

Fig. 214

Type of Treatment: Mobilization with impulse
Goal: Improvement of rotation (right) in the thoracic spine
Technique: Rotation manipulation – shearing hand movement
Therapeutic Usefulness: Great: SWI, SWE, FIN
Moderate: CZE
None: FRG

Procedure: The patient is prone and the thoracic kyphosis is exaggerated. In this example, the operator's right pisiforme bone is placed over the transverse process of, i.e. T9 on the right side. The other hand, facing the opposite direction, is placed over the transverse process of the next inferior vertebral unit (Fig. 215).
The impulse is directed through both transverse processes in an anterior direction.

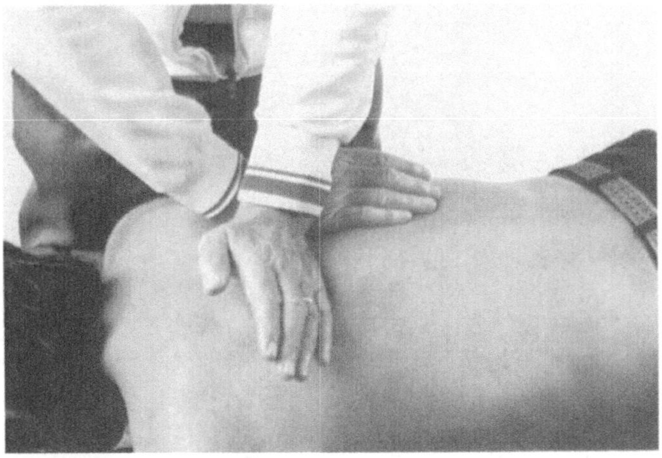

Fig. 215

Type of Treatment: Mobilization with impulse
Goal: To improve rotation of the thoracic spine and mobilization of ribs
Technique: Manipulation to improve rotation
Therapeutic Usefulness: Moderate: USA, SWI, FRG, CZE
None: F

Procedure: With the patient prone, thoracic kyphosis is further accentuated. In this example, the operator's pisiform bone of the left hand is placed over the right transverse process of T5. The pisiforme bone of the right hand is placed over the transverse process of T6 as well as the left sixth rib (Fig. 216).
Both hands introduce the impulse directed anteriorly.

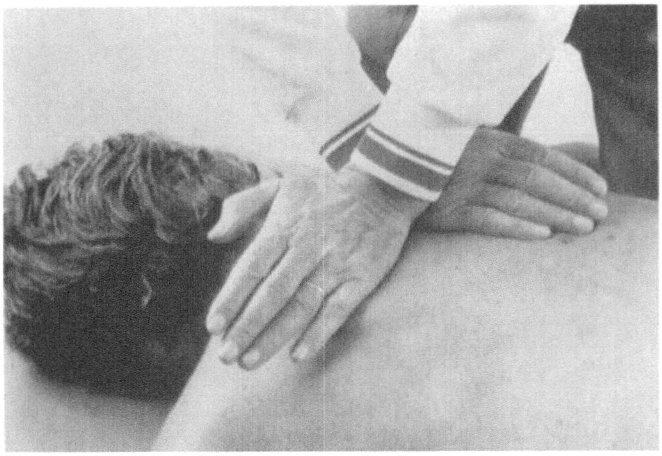

Fig. 216

Type of Treatment: Mobilization with impulse
Goal: Improvement of rotation in the lower thoracic spine
Technique: Rotation manipulation
Therapeutic Usefulness: Great: USA
Procedure: The patient is in the lateral recumbant position with the lumbar and thoracic spine slightly flexed and rotated. The restricted vertebral unit is localized and brought to its barrier (Fig. 217).
The impulse is made through the operator's forearm on the ilium effecting a rotatory motion of the trunk and ilium. The movement is monitored by the operator's fingers at the interspinous interval.

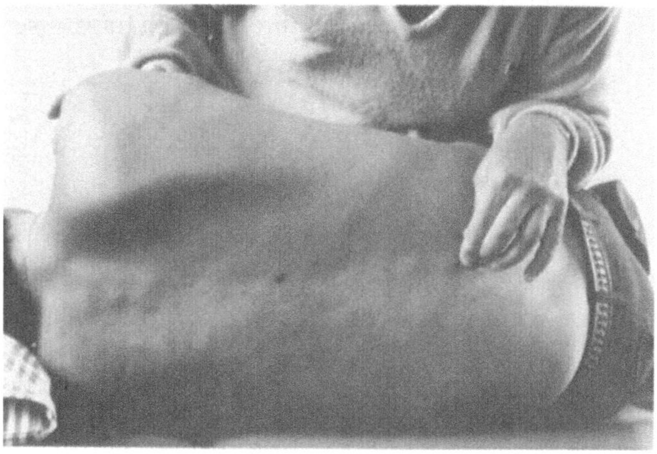

Fig. 217

Type of Treatment: Mobilization with impulse
Goal: Improvement of rotation at the thoraco-lumbar junction
Technique: Rotation manipulation
Therapeutic Usefulness: Great: USA
None: FRG, CZE, SWE, SWI, FIN
Procedure: The patient is prone and his pelvis is stabilized by securing it to the examination table with a belt. The lumbar and thoracic spine are rotated to one side (i.e., right). The thoracic spinous process (T11, for instance) is stabilized with the left hand. The patient's shoulder rests on the operator's sternum (Fig. 218). The impulse is directed towards the right side and follows rotation over the patient's right shoulder.

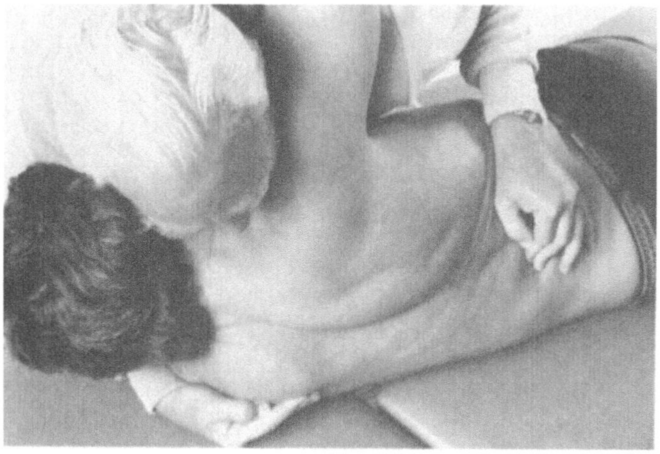

Fig. 218

Type of Treatment: Mobilization with impulse
Goal: Improvement of rotation in the thoraco-lumbar junction
Technique: Rotation manipulation
Therapeutic Usefulness: Great: FRG, USA, SWE, CZE, UK
None: SWI
Procedure: The patient is sitting astride the examination table. Rotation in the vertebral column is introduced through the shoulder girdle (in this example to the left side). The lower thoracic and lumbar spine are flexed and sidebent to the right. The operator's right thumb palpates the right side of the patient's spinous process of L1. The impulse is directed towards the right (Fig. 219).

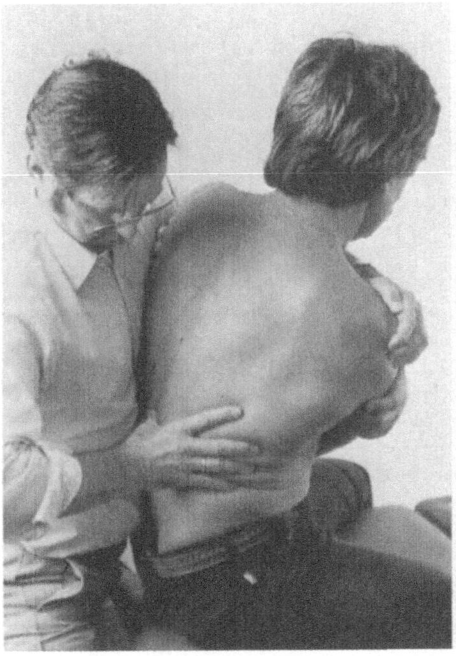

Fig. 219

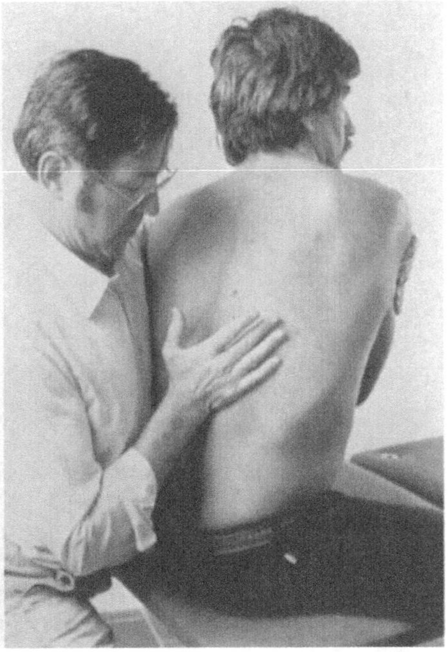

Fig. 220

Type of Treatment: Mobilization with impulse
Goal: Improvement of rotation in the thoraco-lumbar junction
Technique: Manipulation to improve rotation
Therapeutic Usefulness: Great: USA, SWE, FIN, FRG, CZE, SWI
None: UK
Procedure: The patient is seated astride the examination table. The vertebral column is brought to its barrier (in this example through rotation to the left, slight extension at the lumbar spine and sidebending to the left). Through the pisiform bone the operator applies the impulse to the transverse process of T12 following the direction of shoulder rotation (Fig. 220).

Type of Treatment: Mobilization with impulse
Goal: Improvement of rib mobility (Ribs II–VI)
Technique: Rib manipulation
Therapeutic usefulness: Great: FRG
Moderate: SWI, USA
Little: no further information available
Procedure: Treatment is commenced by having the patient in the side-lying recumbant position. In this example, the operator places the left thenar eminence over the restricted rib. The patient is then stabilized in the supine position and rotated slightly to the right (Fig. 221). The impulse is effected through the patient's flexed arms and shoulder girdle (Fig. 222).

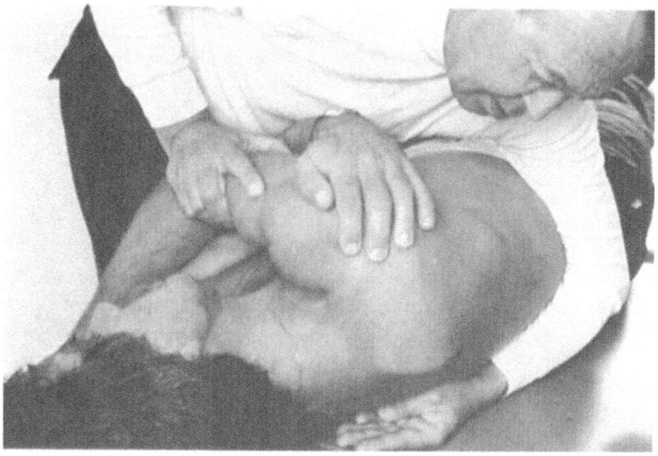

Fig. 221

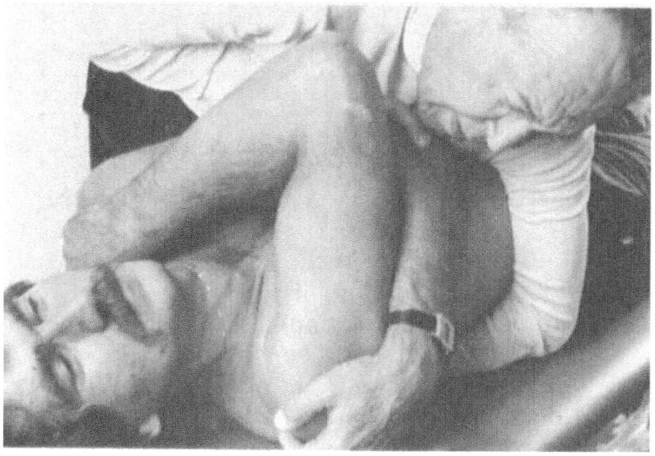

Fig. 222

Type of Treatment: Mobilization with impulse
Goal: Improvement of rib mobility (inferior to and including rib 4)
Technique: Rib manipulation
Therapeutic Usefulness: Great: FRG, FIN
Moderate: SWI, SWE
None: CZE
Procedure: With the patient prone, slight flexion is introduced in the thoracic spine. In this example, the operator's left hypothenar eminence stabilizes the patient's transverse processes of T4–T6). The right hypothenar eminence is placed over the costal angle of the fifth rib (Fig. 213).
The impulse is in an anterior, lateral, and inferior direction.

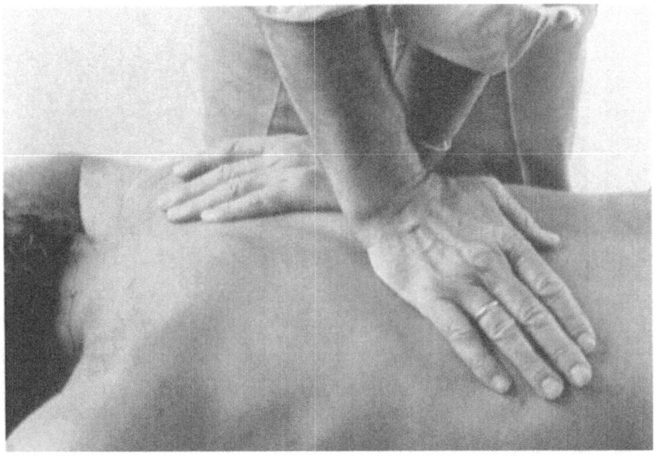

Fig. 223

Type of Treatment: Mobilization with impulse
Goal: Improvement of rib mobility (inferior to and including rib 4)
Technique: Rib manipulation
Therapeutic Usefulness: Great: SWI
None: FRG, USA, F
Procedure: The patient is in the lateral recumbant position. The operator's left middle finger is placed over the costal angle of rib 6, for instance. The operator's right hand provides additional force (Fig. 224). The impulse is in the anterior, lateral, and inferior direction.

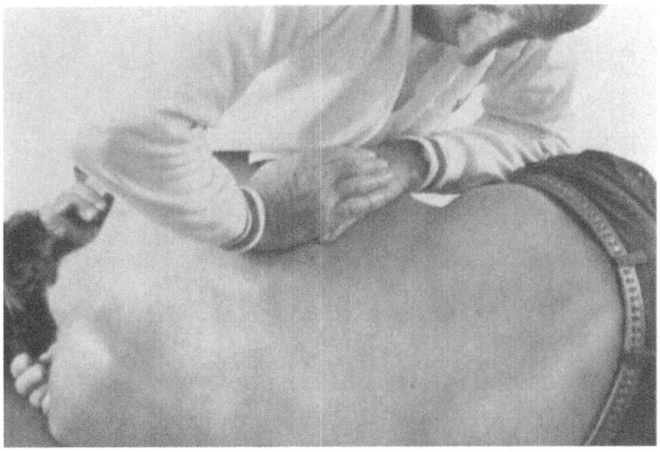

Fig. 224

Type of Treatment: Mobilization with impulse
Goal: Improvement of mobility (central and lower ribs)
Technique: Rib manipulation
Therapeutic Usefulness: Great: no information provided
None: FRG
Procedure: The patient is prone. The operator's hypothenar is placed over the left tenth rib, for example. The operator places his hand flat over a major region of the pelvis (left) and introduces right rotation with his other hand in the lumbar spine until reaching the restricted barrier (Fig. 225). The impulse directed posteriorly is effected through the pelvis with the ribs being stabilized in the opposite direction.

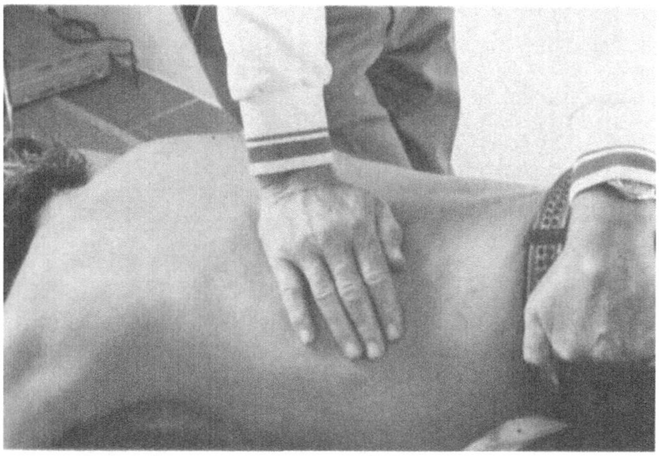

Fig. 225

Type of Treatment: Mobilization with impulse
Goal: Improvement of rib mobility during respiration (inferior to and including rib IV)
Technique: Rib manipulation
Therapeutic Usefulness: Great: F
None: USA, SWI, SWE, FRG
Procedure: The seated patient leans against the operator's thigh.
The operator's fingertips palpate the ribs (Fig. 226).
The impulse is directed either inferiorly or superiorly during exhalation.

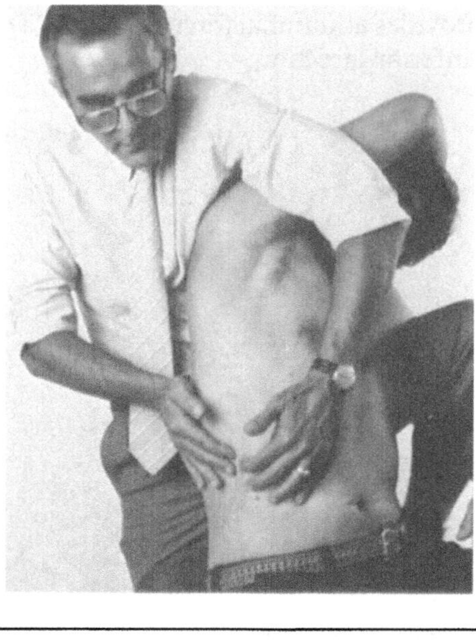

Fig. 226

5.3.4 Muscle Rehabilitation

Type of Treatment: Muscle stretching utilizing post-isometric relaxation
Goal: To stretch the pectoralis major muscle
Technique: Muscle stretch technique
Therapeutic Usefulness: Great: CZE, SWI
Procedure: The patient's arm is abducted and elevated. The operator places one hand flat over the thorax and the other at the elbow of the abducted arm. Isometric contraction of the pectoralis major muscle follows. The pectoralis major muscle is then stretched during the relaxation phase by abducting the arm further and applying simultaneous fine traction (Fig. 227).

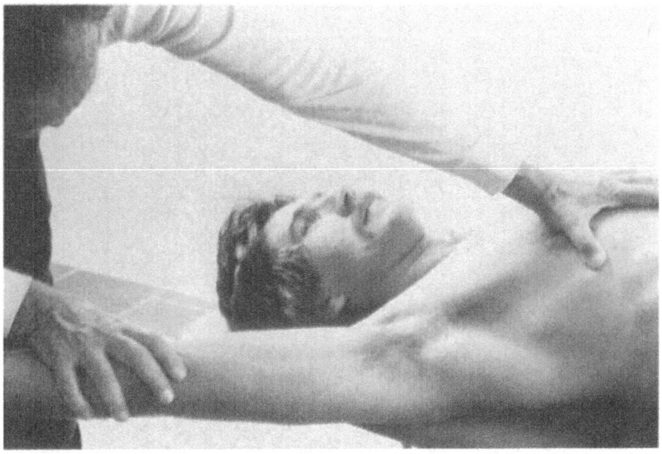

Fig. 227

Type of Treatment: Muscle stretching without utilization of postisometric relaxation
Goal: Lengthening of the erector spinae muscles in the thoracic region
Technique: Muscle stretch techniques
Therapeutic Usefulness: Great: USA, SWE, FRG
Little: SWI
Procedure: The patient is in the lateral recumbant position. The operator's fingers are placed over the thoracic erector muscles. The operator leans with his elbows on the patient's axilla and pelvis (Fig. 228).
Force is applied to the pelvis and thorax in an inferior and superior direction. Sidebending is increased by applying stretch to the erector spinae muscles in the thoracic region.

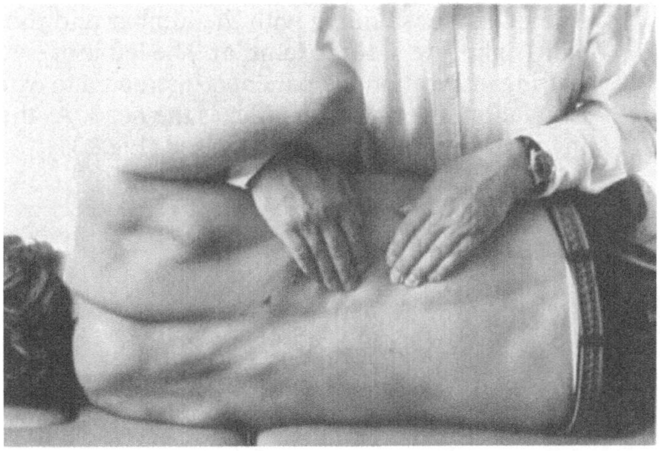

Fig. 228

Type of Treatment: Muscle stretching utilization of post-isometric relaxation
Goal: Stretching of the erector spinae muscles in the thoracic region (i.e., on the left side)
Technique: Muscle stretch technique
Therapeutic Usefulness: Great: CZE, SWI
Procedure: The patient is seated with his hands clasped behind his neck. The thoracic spine is rotated to the right. The patient's inhalation motion is monitored while he rotates the neck and head to the left side, as in this example. This is followed by exhalation and rotation of the head and neck to the right.
The erector spinae muscles are stretched during exhalation by applying additional passive right rotation to the thoracic spine (Fig. 229).

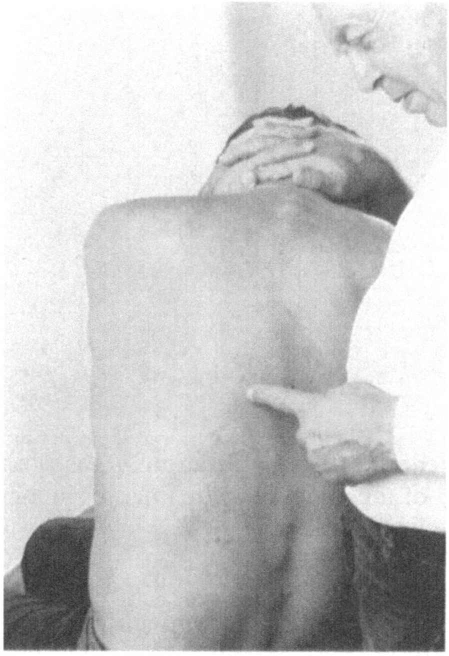

Fig. 229

Type of Treatment: Muscle stretching utilizing post-isometric relaxation
Goal: Stretching of the quadratus lumborum muscle
Technique: Muscle stretch technique
Therapeutic Usefulness: Great: CZE, SWI
Procedure: The patient is standing with the lumbar and thoracic spine sidebent to one side (right side in this example). The left arm is elevated (Fig. 230).
During inspiration the patient is instructed to extend the head. With the next exhalation motion he then flexes the head. As the patient exhales, sidebending in the lumbar spine is increased (Fig. 231).

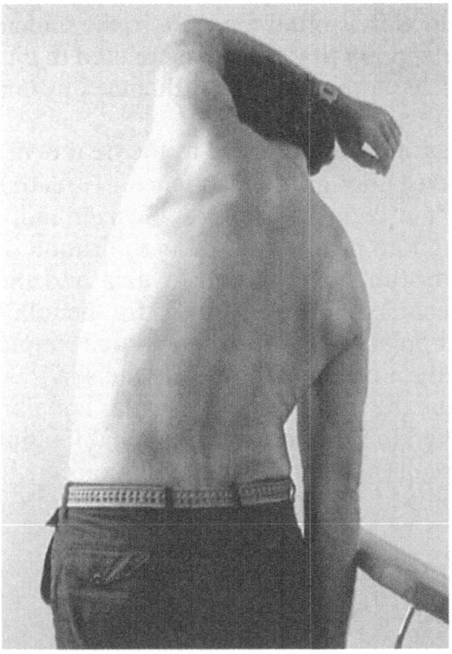

Fig. 230

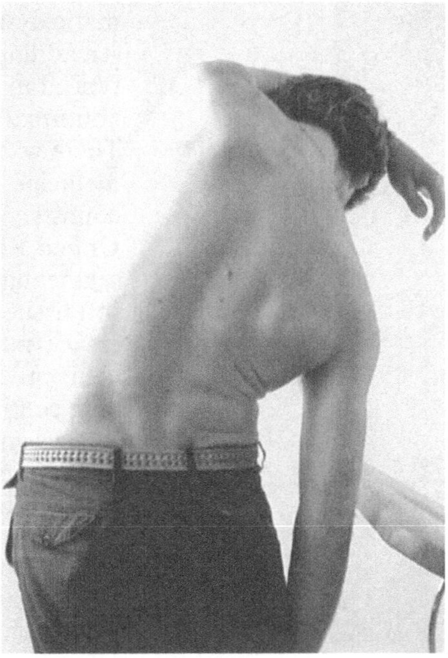

Fig. 231

5.4 Summary

One of the points the group considered important was the difference between the terms mobilization and manipulation. These terms are used differently in the different countries and have been described in the "Terminology" section of the book (Chap. 1).

There was agreement that diagnosis should consist of a complete history followed by an overall assessment, a physical and structural examination of the axial skeleton and the extremities before proceeding with the segmental examination. The different schools agreed, that in no case is it sufficient to examine only those painful regions indicated by the patient.

The representatives from the Scandinavian countries, in particular, emphasized the use of gross motion testing as a part of the diagnostic procedure. Soft tissues including the different muscles are examined by palpation as well as functional evaluation. The purpose of this examination is to elicit regions with segmental dysfunctions and their respective restricted motions, as emphasized by the osteopathic physicians. The French and Swiss schools utilized specific procedures to provoke pain in the patient as a part of diagnosis emphasizing the importance of zones of irritations. The Czechoslavakian representative emphasized the use of general motion patterns during diagnosis, such as functionally related muscle groups, especially shortened postural muscles and weakened phasic muscles that present as muscular imbalances.

The recognition of viscero-somatic reflexes was felt to be very important clinically and thus formed a significant aspect of diagnosis in the axial skeleton. The identification of viscero-somatic reflexes is not only used in the diagnosis and differential diagnosis but is also of concern in patients with

visceral disease such as myocardial infarction on angina pectoris, where somatic dysfunction is often manifest in the mid and upper thoracic spine.
An additional point that was made related to diagnosis was that posture and typical muscle patterns can be influenced by emotional problems as well as abnormal breathing.
There was agreement in regard to the treatment procedures used in manual medicine, even though the sequence of treatment varied from country to country. While countries such as Switzerland, Germany, France, and the United Kingdom primarily used mobilization or manipulation to resolve a segmental dysfunction, Czechoslovakia and the USA employed primarily soft tissue techniques as preparation for the following mobilization or, if necessary, manipulation. Those schools that employ manipulation as a treatment procedure of choice integrate the services of physical therapists who then continue the treatment of muscular imbalance. The physical therapist's role was noted in the context of the rehabilitation process.
The participants agreed that manipulations are to be limited both in number and duration without, however, setting the upper limits in exact numbers.

Chapter 6

Lumbar Spine and Sacroiliac Joints

Participants:
Italy (I): G. Brugnoni
Sweden (SWE): I. Hamberg
Switzerland (SWI): U. Waller
USA: P. Greenman and S. Haldeman
West Germany (FRG): H. D. Neumann

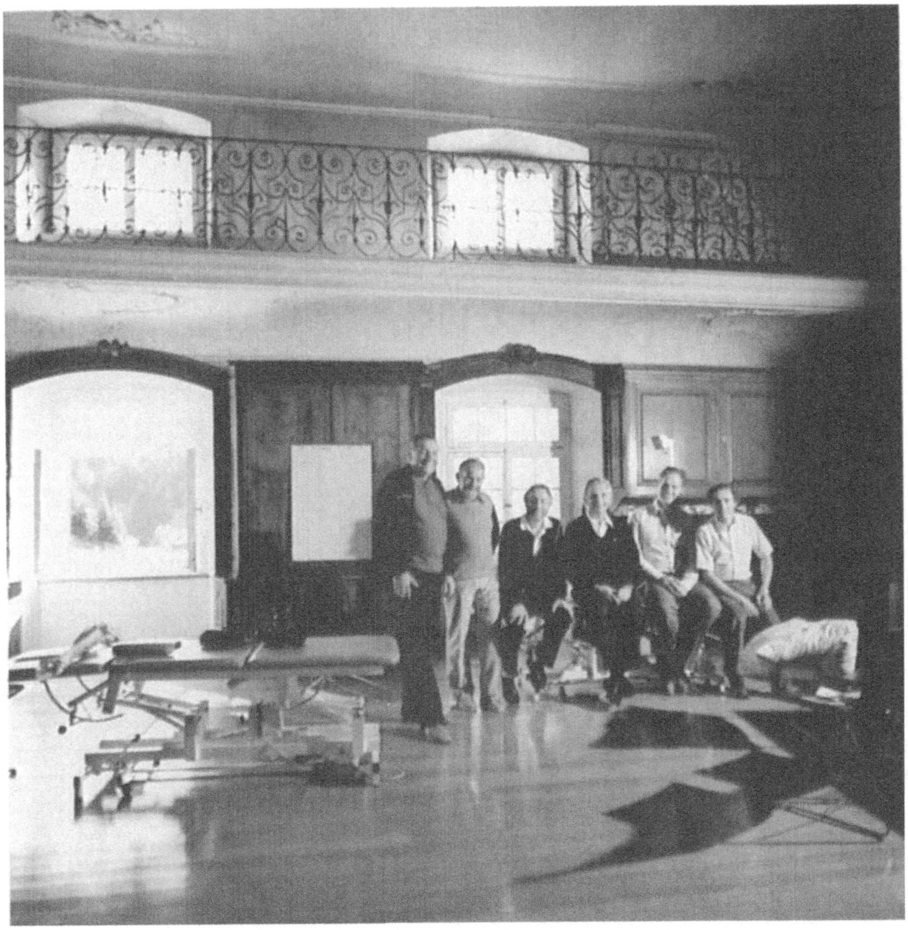

6.1 Biomechanics of the Lumbar Spine, Lumbo-Sacral Junction and Sacroiliac Joints

The smallest functional unit of the spine is the spinal segment, which is comprised of the following:

1. Structures Involved in Motion
   - intervertebral disk
   - apophyseal joint
2. Structures Responsible for Stabilization
   - ligaments
   - joint capsule

Motion in the Lumbar Spine

As a result of the orientation of the joint surfaces, the major motions that are possible in the lumbar spine are those of flexion and extension (Fig. 232), whereas rotation about the Y- and Z-axis is a coupled motion.

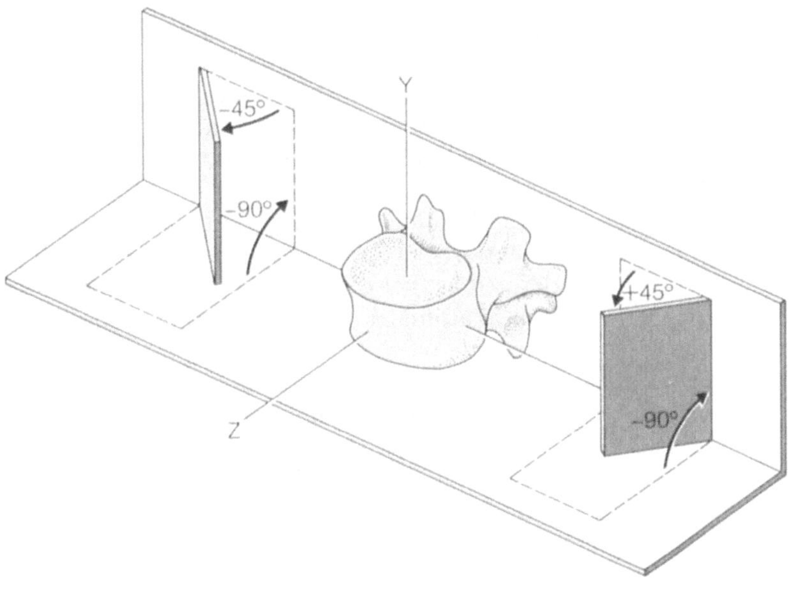

Fig. 232. Graphical representation of the facet joint inclinations and axes of motion of a lumbar vertebra (After White and Panjabi 1978)

Sidebending and rotation motions are always coupled. When the lumbar spine is flexed, the coupled motions of sidebending and rotation are in the same direction, whereas with the spine extended the they are in the opposite directions (Fig. 233).

There was general agreement as to the underlying mechanisms. It is the Italian representative's opinion, however, that rotation is impossible when the lumbar spine is extended since the apophyseal joints are in a locked position thereby preventing rotation. The osteopathic representative from the USA noted that there is only minimal rotation when the lumbar spine is extended.

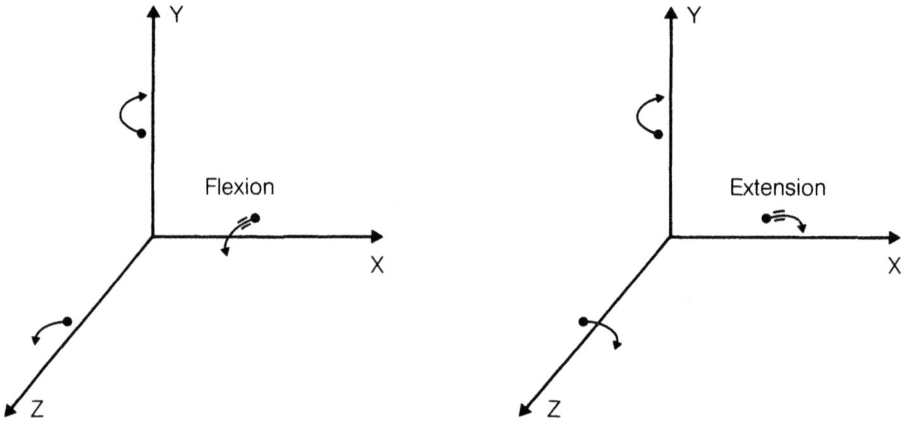

Fig. 233. Coupling patterns seen in the lumbar spine during flexion

Sacroiliac Joints

- The flexion and extension motions of the sacrum are described as a nutation type of movement (Fig. 234).
- Sacral Movement During the Walking Cycle. The movement occurring during the walking cycle is such that rotation and sidebending are to opposite directions, and there is an anterior nutational component to one side of the base of the sacrum.
  The anterior surface will rotate to the left, the sacral base will decline to the right, and the base will move anteriorly resulting in the Figure 8 movement.
- Iliac Movement. During the walking cycle, the ilia rotate anteriorly and posteriorly, in an opposing fashion. Anterior and posterior movements are defined as that direction in which the superior aspect of the crest travels. The anatomical and palpatory landmark is the posterior superior iliac spine.
  Furthermore, the crest of the ilium moves somewhat superiorly and laterally, while the ischium moves postero-medially.

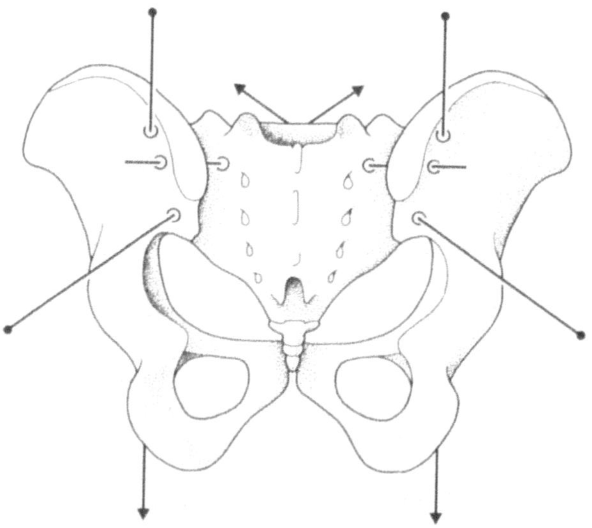

Fig. 234. Axes of motion in the sacroiliac joints

Other movements associated with the sacroiliac joints include:
- The motion described by Lewit as "gapping." The American terms are "inflare" and "outflare."
- In addition, there can exist a superior-inferior shear movement of the ilia, which is primarily seen in patients with parallel and "flat" sacroiliac joints. The sacroiliac joint undergoes nonphysiological movement when the trunk is flexed and simultaneously sidebent. This leads to a posterior nutational movement of the sacrum with rotation to the opposite side, resulting in a strained joint and a dysfunctional position. Furthermore, the adaptive property of the lumbar spine to respond to sacral motion is altered.

Movement of the Pubis

- During the walking cycle there is an anterior and posterior torsional movement which occurs alternately between the right and left pubic bone. This motion appears to be about a horizontal axis.
- In single leg standing, there is a superior to inferior shear movement which occurs along a vertical axis.

Coupled Lumbar – Sacral Movement

During the walking cycle, there is coupled lumbar and sacral movement, in opposite directions, however. That is, when the sacrum sidebends to the right and rotates to the left, L_5 rotates to the right. This mechanism is the result of the function of the iliolumbar ligaments (Fig. 235).

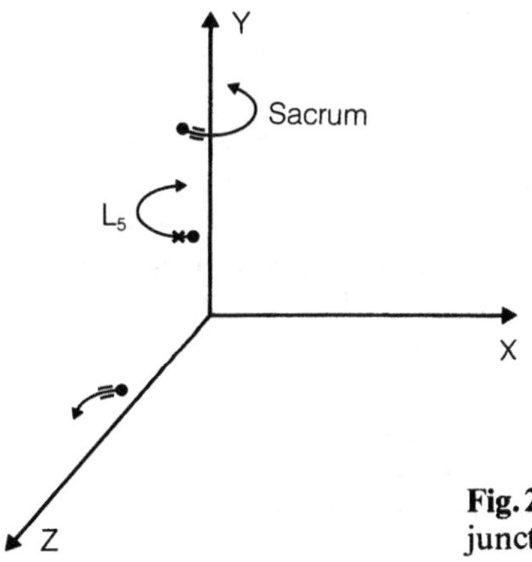

Fig. 235. Coupling patterns seen in the lumbosacral junction

6.2 Diagnosis

6.2.1 Diagnostic Criteria for the Lumbar Spine, Lumbo-Sacral Junction and Sacroiliac Joints

6.2.1.1 Functional Disorders

1. Motion Restriction in Contrast to Normal Mobility or Hypermobility.
The Italian school believes that one cannot palpate the range of motion of an individual vertebra by way of the spinous process. One of the criteria for restricted motion is the so-called "joint play."
2. Altered Tissue Texture (Static Palpation)
- muscles
- ligaments
- fascia
- subcutaneous tissue
- skin
3. Provocative Testing
4. Muscular Imbalance

Regarding the assessment of functional disturbances, specific consideration is given to:
- Motion Restriction
  - gross motion
  - multisegmental mobility
  - unisegmental mobility
  - active mobility
  - passive mobility
  - resisted motion
- Altered Tissue Texture (Static Palpation)
  - Skin: Kibler skin-fold, or skin-drag, temperature, color, tension, smoothness
  - subcutaneous tissue: bogginess, edema, tension
  - fascia: movement (ease and bind)
  - muscles including the muscle-tendon junction, tendons
  - hyper- and hypotonus, trigger points, contractions and fibrotic changes
  - ligaments: tension (tightness-relaxed), pain, fibrotic changes
  - segmental zones of irritation
- Provocative Tests (dynamic palpation)
  - pain on joint movement
  - tissue reaction on movement
  multisegmental, or unisegmental
  active and passive
  - pain on joint pressure (French school)
  - joint play
  - zone of irritation (Swiss school)
- Imbalance Tests (static and dynamic)
  - gait
  - posture: left-right
    anterior-posterior
    superior-inferior
  - muscles: shortening of the postural muscle groups
    weakening of phasic muscle groups

6.2.1.2 *Prognostic Factors*

Factors associated with a poor prognosis
- postural imbalance
- muscular imbalance
- hypermobility
  - acquired
  - constitutional
- psychosomatic disturbances
  - tension
  - stress
  - depression
- duration of the functional disorder
- poor general health

Factors associated with a good prognosis
- a skillful physician
- good patient cooperation
- short time of onset and short duration
- one-directional motion restriction
- insignificant, minimal soft tissue alteration, i.e., edema, fibrosis, muscle-tension, vascular changes
- isolated muscle weakening or shortening of one single muscle.

6.2.2 Tissue Texture Examination

Spinal Area: Lumbar spine
Type of Examination: Layer palpation
Diagnostic Usefulness: Great: SWI, USA, I, SWE
Moderate: FRG

Procedure: The fingertips of the palpating finger rest broadly over the individual segment (Fig. 236). The following structures are evaluated in order: skin, fascia, muscles, joint capsule, periosteum (bone).
Smoothness, resistance, pain upon pressure and resistance to movement in the individual layers are evaluated.

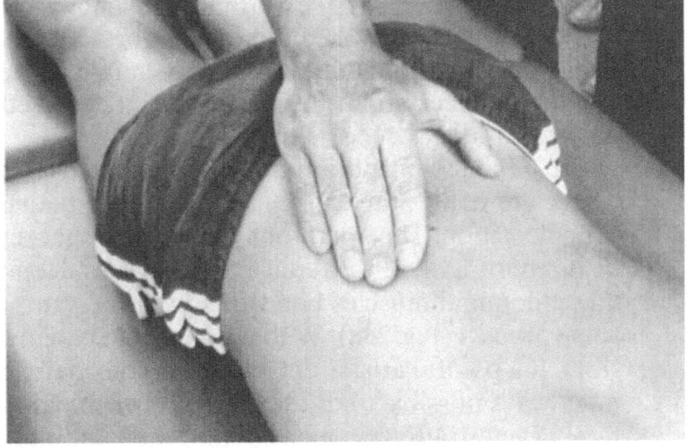

Fig. 236

Spinal Area: Lumbar spine
Type of Examination: Palpation of the cutaneaus and subcutaneous tissues
Diagnostic Usefulness: Moderate: FRG, I, SWE
None: USA, SWI

Procedure: Both hands form a skinfold with thumb and index finger (Fig. 237) which is followed inferiorly ("pincer rouler").
Evaluated are:
1. changes in skin thickness,
2. pain.

Each dermatome correlates with one vertebral unit, which in contrast, however, does not correlate with metamere consequences.

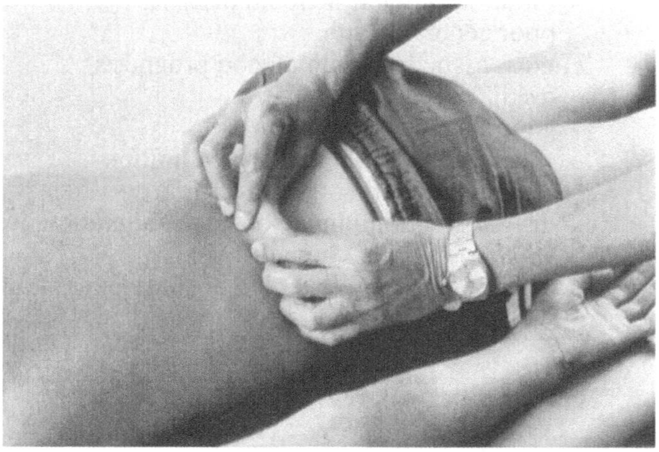

Fig. 237

Spinal Area: Lumbar spine and sacroiliac joints
Type of Examination: Zone of irritation evaluation
Diagnostic Usefulness: Great: SWI
Moderate: SWE? USA, I
None: FRG

Procedure: The following different tissue texture abnormalities are found by palpation of the musculoskeletal system:
1. an immovable "doughy" edema.
2. tissue texture abnormalities sometimes found close to the joint capsule, as well as over the sacroiliac joint at the neighboring bony structures (such as the sacrum itself).
3. provocative testing is performed. The pain is compounded when provocative testing is in the direction of the dysfunction and decreases when moved away from the dysfunction. Pain completely disappears if manipulation is successful or if the problem is resolved.
4. systematic sequence.

In the lumbar spine, the zones of irritation that are located at the costal processes are of of practical importance. The patient rests comfortably in the prone position. The operator's palpating finger reaches around the iliocostalis lumborum muscle laterally, then presses deeply between this muscle and the abdominal muscles beneath so that he can palpate the tip of the transverse process (Fig. 238). With a non-obese patient bone contact is easily possible. If a painful area is detected, it is considered pathological. It is however not always possible to differentiate between painful tendinoses of the lateral lumbar intertransverse muscles and the quadratus lumborum muscle.

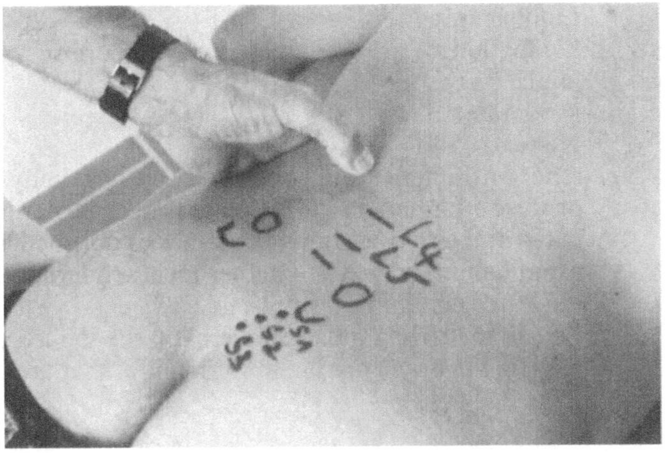

Fig. 238

The zones of irritation are palpated at the lateral margin of the inferior pole of the spinous process. Due to their close proximity to the mamillary processes and the corresponding insertions of the transverse-spinal and sacrospinal muscles, the zones of irritation located at the superior articular processes cannot always be directly identified.

The zones of irritation in the sacroiliac joint region are palpated at the lateral sacral crest between the posterior inferior iliac spine and the sacral horn. The zone of irritation of S1 is located 1 cm medially to the posterior inferior iliac spine while the zone of irritation correlating with S3 is proximal to the sacral horn with the zone of irritation of S2 lying between these two (Fig. 239). The free margin of the sacrum is identified, and the palpating thumb presses down between the erector spinae muscles and the gluteus maximus muscle so as to reach the deep bony portion of the sacrum.

The zone of irritation at the sacroiliac joint often disappears when pressure is applied to the sacrum in an anterior direction. This can be accomplished through the hypothenar eminence of the nonpalpating hand. When the hypothenar eminence ceases to provide pressure, a stabbing pain becomes apparent. The palpating thumb must rest with constant pressure over the zone of irritation while anterior pressure is maintained.

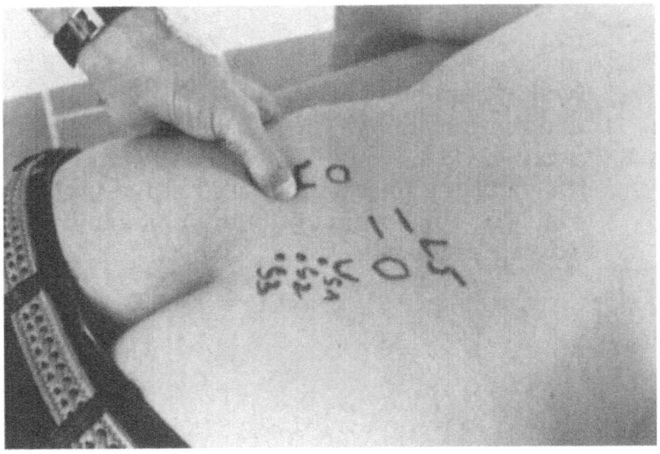

Fig. 239

Spinal Area:	Lumbar spine
Type of Examination:	Evaluation of areas tender upon pressure in the region of the apophyseal joints
Diagnostic Usefulness:	Moderate: SWI, I None: FRG, USA, SWE
Procedure:	After pushing the longissimus muscles medially and laterally the mamillary process is palpated. The articular process superior to this process is then palpated and as close a bony contact is established as is possible (Fig. 240). This examination evaluates whether local tenderness and/or pain radiating into the lower extremities is present.
Remarks:	Due to the strong muscles overlying the joint capsules it is often difficult to palpate the tissue texture abnormalities that are related to it.

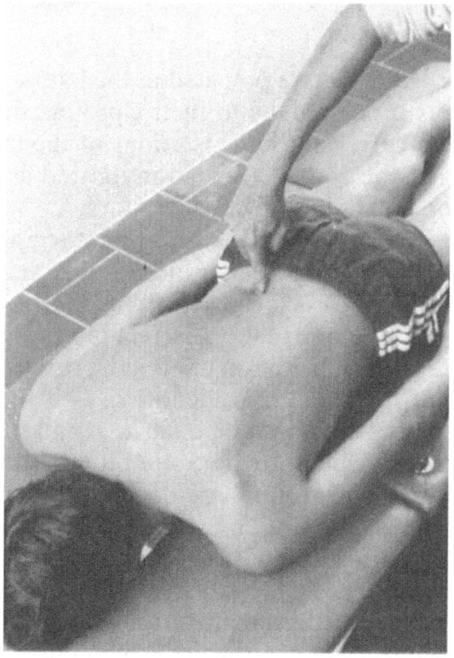

Fig. 240

6.2.3 Motion Testing

Spinal Area:	Symphysis pubis
Type of Examination:	Static examination of the pubic bone and related tenderness
Diagnostic Usefulness:	Great: I, USA, SWI, FRG, SWE
Procedure:	The palpating fingers are placed at the superior border of the pubic bone (Fig. 241). The position of both pubic rami towards each other and tender areas are evaluated.

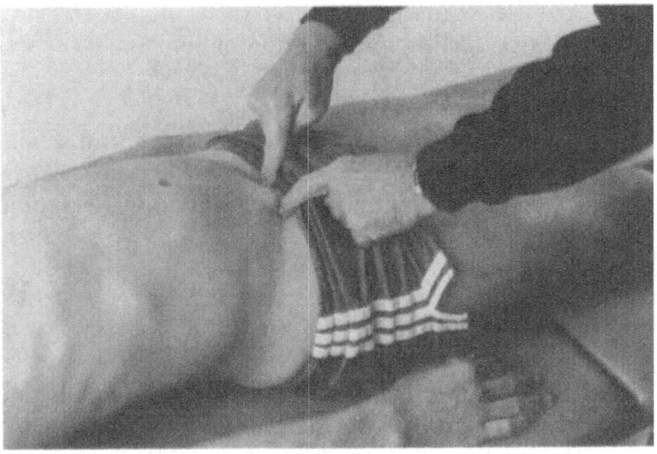

Fig. 241

Spinal Area: Lumbar spine

Type of Examination: Lumbar flexion evaluation

Diagnostic Usefulness:
Great: I
Moderate: SWI, USA, SWE
None: FRG, USA

Procedure: With the arms locked in front of the body, the patient internally rotates his feet and bends forward maximally (Fig. 242). Evaluated are:

1. restriction of motion in the sagittal direction,
2. pain,
3. changes of the thoraco-lumbar junction in the frontal plane during flexion (greater or less scoliosis formation),
4. changes in motion patterns of the thoracosacral junction (vertebral column motion in relationship to the hip bone).

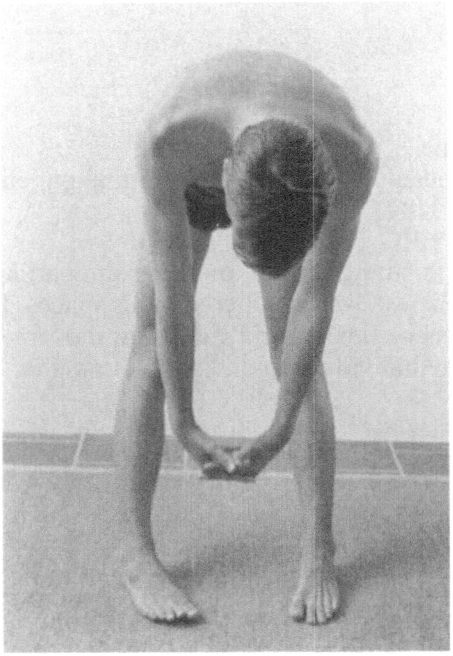

Fig. 242

Spinal Area: Lumbar spine
Type of Examination: Flexion testing in the sitting patient
Diagnostic Usefulness: Great: USA, FRG
Moderate: SWI, SWE

Procedure: The operator's thumbs rest over the transverse processes of one segment. The patient is instructed to slowly bend forward while the operator evaluates quality and symmetry of the individual segments.

Spinal Area: Lumbar spine
Type of Examination: Flexion testing in the supine patient
Diagnostic Usefulness: Great: FRG, SWI
Moderate: USA, SWE

Procedure: In the lateral recumbant position, the patient's hip and knees are flexed. The examiner introduces flexion with the free hand in the vertebral column by flexing the patient's thighs (Fig. 243). With the other hand the operator palpates the lumbar spinous processes and the interspinous distance which normally increases during this procedure.

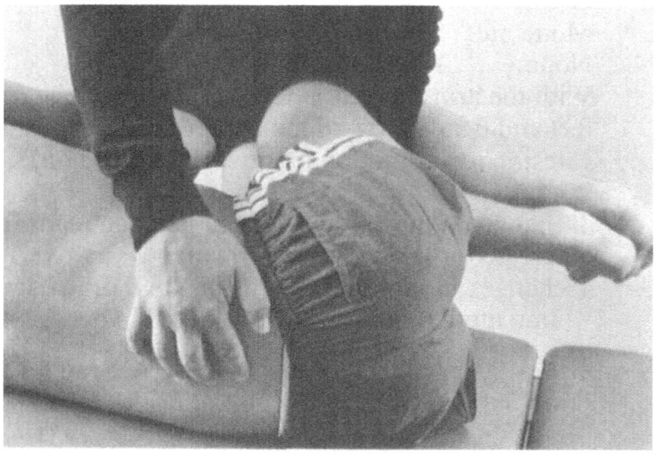

Fig. 243

Spinal Area: Lumbar spine
Type of Examination: Flexion-extension evaluation in the sitting patient
Diagnostic Usefulness: Great: USA
Moderate: FRG, SWI, SWE

Procedure: The patient is sitting upright on the examination table. The operator's palpating fingers rest over the inter-spinous spaces. The operator's free hand introduces passive flexion and extension movement evaluating the range of motion in the individual spinous processes (Fig. 244).

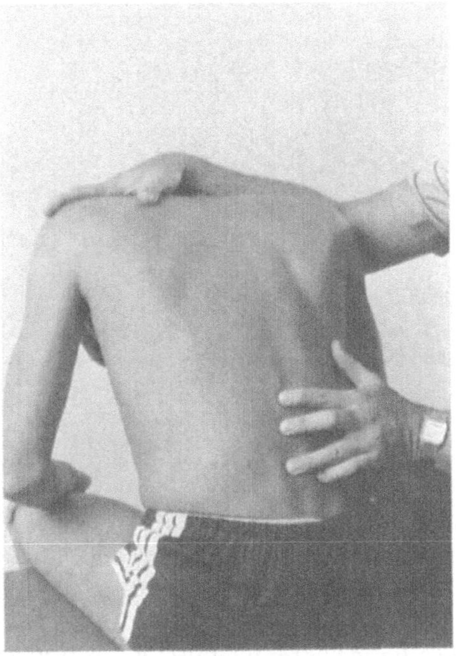

Fig. 244

Spinal Area: Lumbar spine
Type of Examination: Extension evaluation
Diagnostic usefulness: Great: USA, FRG
Moderate: SWI, SWE

Procedure: The patient is prone. The operator's thumbs rest over the articular processes of one segment (Fig. 245). Evaluated is the position of the articular processes in regard to the frontal plane. If one articular process is more posterior it is said that the "the joint cannot open." The patient is then instructed to raise himself on his elbows (extension) and again the symmetry of the position of the individual articular processes is evaluated (Fig. 246).

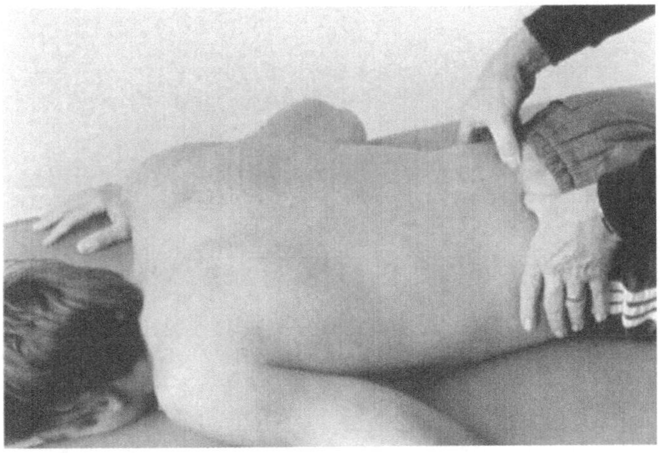

Fig. 245

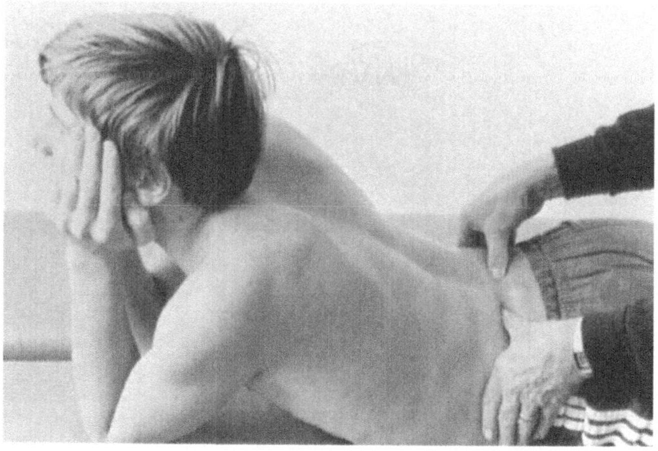

Fig. 246

Spinal Area: Lumbar spine
Type of Examination: Extension evaluation of the lumbar spine
Diagnostic Usefulness: Great: FRG, SWI
Moderate: USA, SWE

Procedure: The patient is in the lateral recumbant position and flexes both hip and knee joints approximately 90°. The operator stabilizes the patient's thighs with one hand while with the other hand he guides the pelvis posteriorly extending the lumbar spine further (Fig. 247). The interspinous distance is evaluated, and should normally decrease during this procedure.

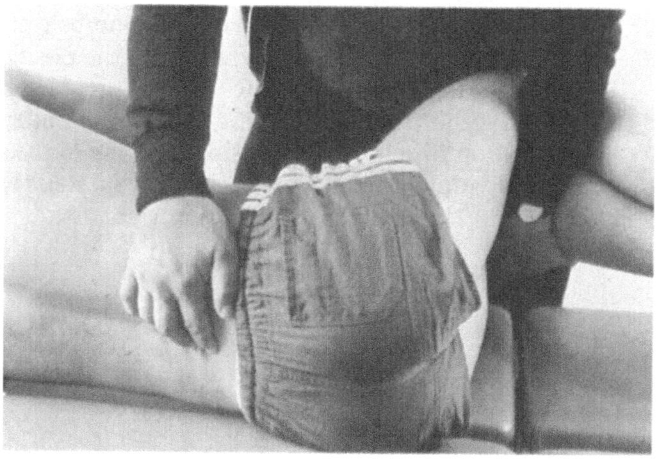

Fig. 247

Spinal Area: Lumbar spine
Type of Examination: Gross motion testing and examination during sidebending
Diagnostic Usefulness: Great: I
Moderate: USA, SWI, SWE
None: FRG

Procedure: The patient, standing with his feet rotated internally, performing active sidebending of the trunk (Fig. 248).
Evaluated are:
1. pain provocation,
2. motion restriction in the frontal plane,
3. multisegmental motion changes.

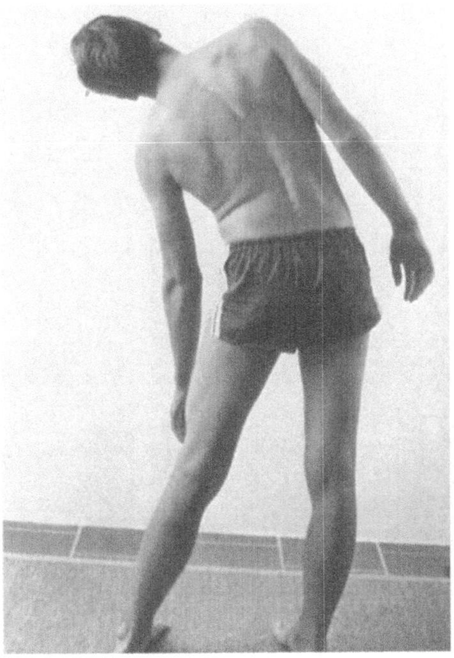

Fig. 248

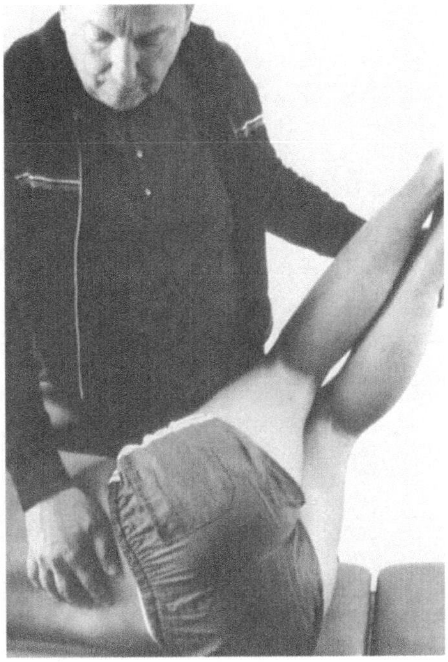

Fig. 249

Spinal Area: Lumbar spine
Type of Examination: Sidebending evaluation
Diagnostic Usefulness: Great: FRG, I
Moderate: USA, SWE

Procedure: In the lateral recumbant position, the patient flexes both hip and knee approximately 90°. The operator's free hand moves the patient's legs and pelvis laterally and superiorly by lifting the patient's feet at the ankles. The patient's thighs rest on one of the operator's thighs (Fig. 249). The palpating hand evaluates if any "sharp dropoffs" between the individual vertebrae are present.

Spinal Area: Lumbar spine
Type of Examination: Evaluation for sidebending and coupled motions
Diagnostic Usefulness: Great: USA
Moderate: FRG, SWI, SWE
Procedure: The patient is sitting on the examination table. With one hand, the operator palpates the interspinous spaces, while the other hand introduces passive sidebending and rotation (Fig. 250). Evaluated are motion of the individual spinous processes.

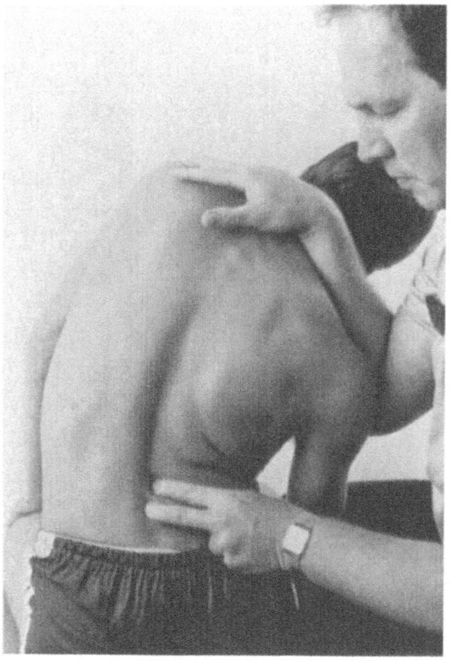
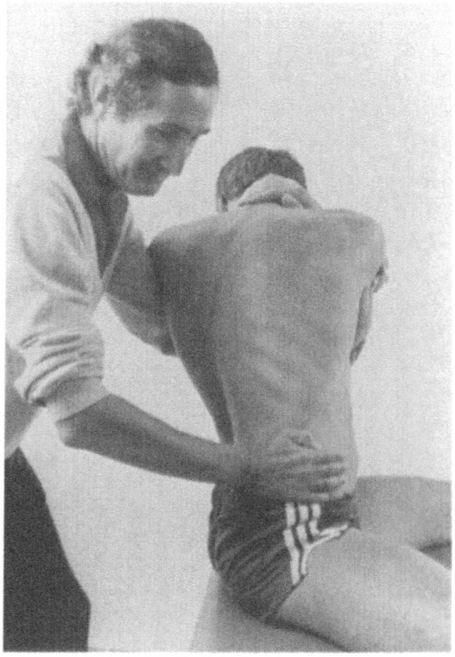

Fig. 250 **Fig. 251**

Spinal Area: Lumbar spine
Type of Examination: Multisegmental rotation
Diagnostic Usefulness: Great: I
Moderate: USA, FRG, SWE, SWI
Procedure: The patient is sitting. The operator places the palm of the hand over the cos-to-transverse processes of the lumbar spine. The other hand introduces maximal passive rotation of the trunk (Fig. 251). In this maneuver, the motion barrier and presence of pain are evaluated.

Spinal Area: Lumbar spine
Type of Examination: Rotation testing
Diagnostic Usefulness: Great: FRG, SWI
Moderate: CZE, USA
Procedure: The patient rests in the right lateral recumbent position. By introducing flexion in the hip and knee joints the patient's superior foot is placed at the calf of the opposite leg. The free hand rotates the pelvis so far as to engage the vertebral motor unit of interest. The palpating finger feels whether the inferior spinous process moves further than the superior spinous process (Fig. 252).

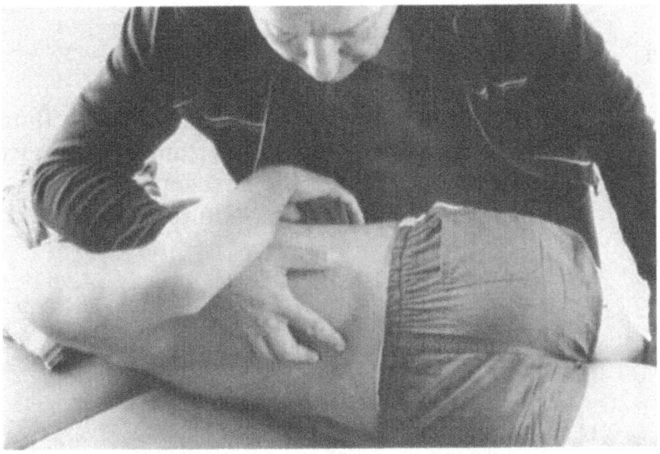

Fig. 252

Spinal Area:	Lumbar spine
Type of Examination:	Joint play and "end feel" evaluation
Diagnostic Usefulness:	Great: USA, SWE
	Moderate: SWI
	None: FRG
Procedure:	The patient is sitting on the examination table. The examiner's thumb is placed over the lateral aspect of the spinous process. The operator's free hand introduces maximal sidebending (Fig. 253). Once in this position, the thumb is pressed laterally on the spinous process allowing the operator to evaluate joint play.

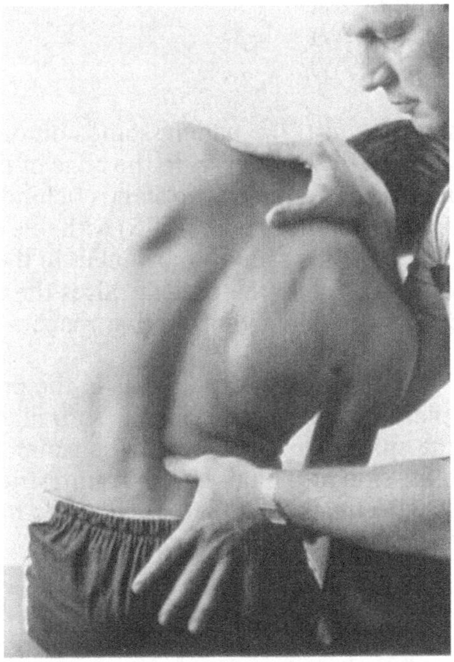

Fig. 253

Spinal Area: Lumbar spine
Type of Examination: Joint play evaluation
Diagnostic Usefulness: Great: I, FRG, SWE, USA, SWI
Procedure: The patient is prone. One of the examiner's thumbs presses laterally on the spinous process while the other thumb presses from the opposite side on the lateral portion of either the next superior or next inferior vertebra (Fig. 254). With a springing type of motion resistance, pain and joint play are evaluated.

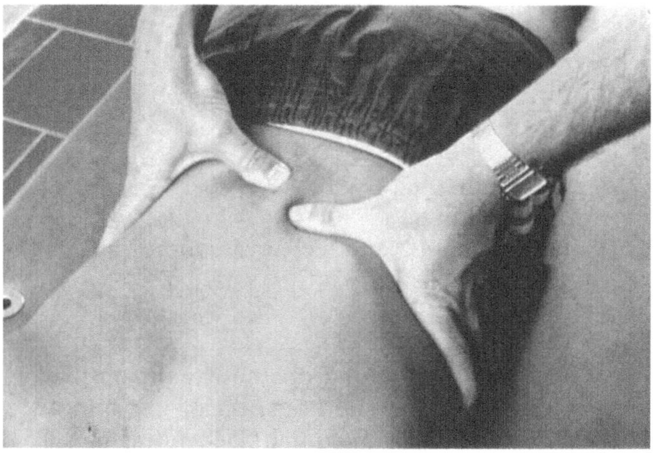

Fig. 254

Spinal Area: Sacroiliac joint
Type of Examination: Single leg standing test
Diagnostic Usefulness: Great: USA, SWI
Moderate: FRG, SWE
None: I
Procedure: Single leg standing test: the patient stands on one leg while balancing himself with one hand by holding on to the edge of the examination table or the back of a chair. The examiner who stands behind the patient's back palpates the posterior superior iliac spine (PSIS) with one hand and monitors with the other hand the patient's sacrum movement in the sacroiliac joint of the side of the standing leg, while the patient raises the opposite leg (which is incidentally flexed at the knee joint) until it reaches the end position in the hip (Fig. 255).
Spine Test: The patient is positioned as in the preceding examination. With one thumb placed over the posterior superior iliac spine and the other thumb resting on the spinous process of S2, the examiner evaluates movement of the PSIS on the side of the raised leg. If unrestricted, the PSIS moves inferiorly whereas when restricted, there is either no movement noted at all or the movement is in a superior direction.

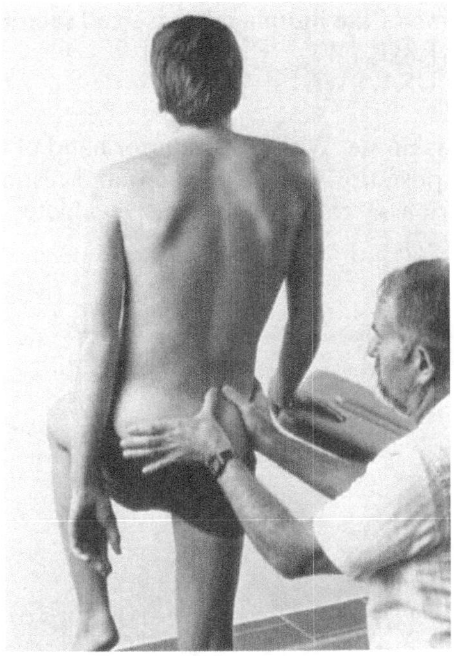

Fig. 255

Spinal Area: Sacroiliac joints
Type of Examination: Standing flexion test
Diagnostic Usefulness: Great: FRG, USA, SWI, SWE
None: I
Procedure: The patient is standing with the feet interacetabular distance apart. The operator who is behind the patient's back palpates with his thumbs the posterior superior iliac spine and instructs the patient to slowly bend forward (Fig. 256). A more pronounced superior movement of the superior posterior iliac spine on one side indicates a dysfunction in the ipsilateral sacroiliac joint. During this maneuver are also noted any changes in symmetry of the lumbar spine, the thorax and ribs, and unilateral muscle contractions (myotendinoses) in the longissimus muscles are evaluated.

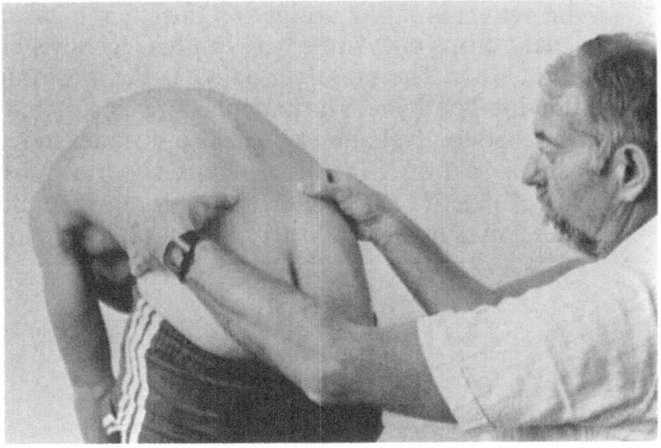

Fig. 256

Spinal Area: Sacroiliac joint
Type of Examination: Motion testing of the ilium against a fixed sacrum
Diagnostic Usefulness: Great: FRG, SWI
Moderate: USA, SWE
None: I
Procedure: The patient is prone. While the anterior hand of the operator guides the patient's ilium posteriorly, the opposite hand resting over the sacrum and the short posterior sacroiliac ligaments, evaluates mobility in the sacroiliac joints (Fig. 257).

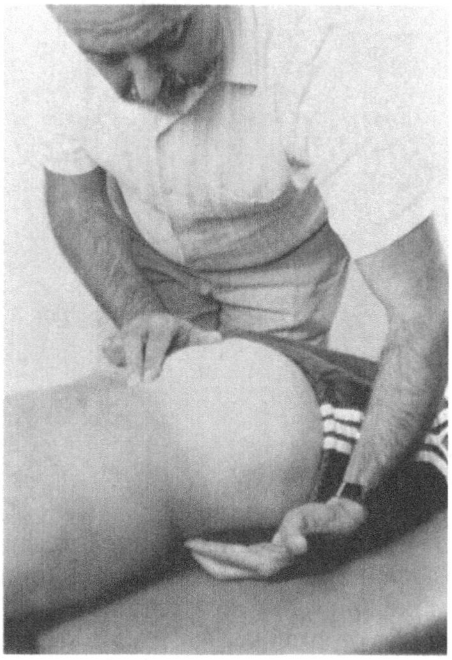

Fig. 257

Spinal Area: Sacroiliac joint
Type of Examination: Seated flexion test
Diagnostic Usefulness: Great: USA, FRG
Moderate: SWI, SWE
Procedure: The patient is sitting upright on the examination table or a stable chair. The patient drops both arms between his legs. It is important that both feet rest on the floor. The examiner palpates the most inferior point of the posterior superior iliac spine. The patient is then instructed to bend forward (Fig. 258). The operator evaluates whether both spines move superiorly in a symmetric fashion or if one side moves more superiorly when compared to the other side. A positive seated flexion test (one spine moves more superiorly) indicates a dysfunction in the ipsilateral sacroiliac joint.

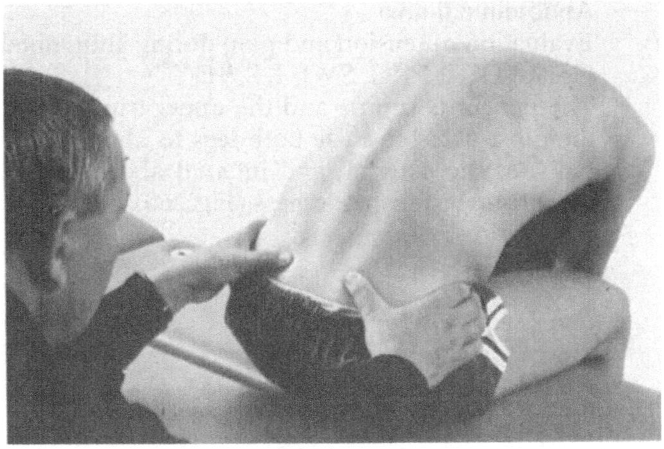

Fig. 258

6.2.4 Neuromuscular Evaluation

Spinal Area: Gluteal Region
Type of Examination: Stretch and provocative testing of the gluteal muscles
Diagnostic Usefulness: Great: USA, FRG, SWI, I, SWE
Procedure: The patient is prone and is instructed to contract one leg isometrically. The contours of the gluteal muscles are evaluated as to symmetry. The muscular insertions are palpated to determine if painful origintendinoses are present (Fig. 259).

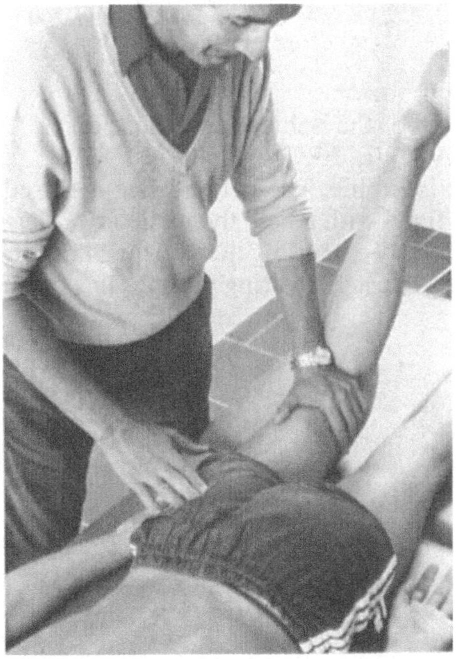

Fig. 259

Spinal Area: Abdomininal area
Type of Examination: Evaluation of tension and pain during abdominal muscle contraction
Diagnostic Usefulness: Great: USA, FRG, SWI, I, SWE
Procedure: The patient is supine and the upper trunk is slightly flexed. The patient is then instructed to raise both legs to about 45°. During this maneuver one palpates the external and internal abdominal oblique muscles examining them for possible tenderness (Fig. 260).

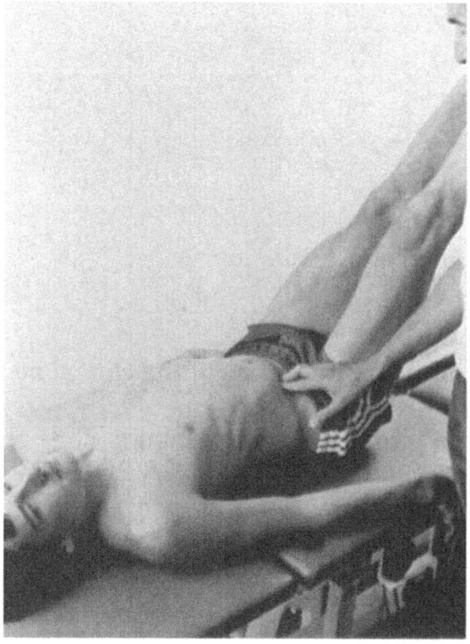

Fig. 260

Spinal Area: Pelvis and hip region
Type of Examination Length testing of the ischio-crural muscles
Diagnostic Usefulness: Great: USA, SWE, FRG, I, SWI
Procedure: The patient is supine. The patient's leg is flexed maximally in the hip joint and is then fixed with a belt, the while lower leg is placed against the operator's shoulder. By extending the patient's knee the operator evaluates whether shortening in the hamstring muscles has occurred (Fig. 261).

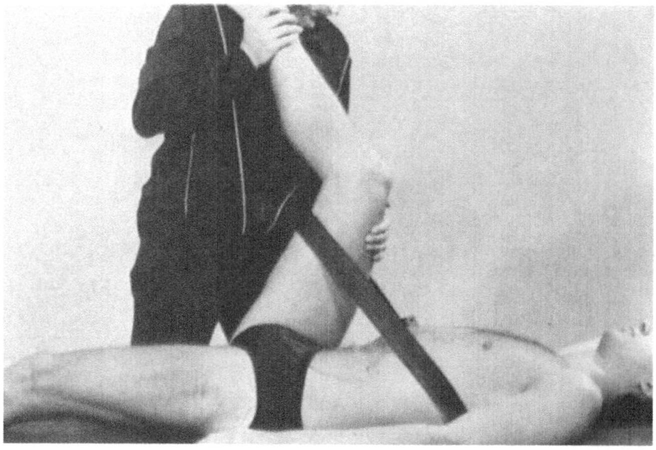

Fig. 261

Spinal Area: Lumbo-sacral junction
Type of Examination: Iliopsoas muscle length testing
Diagnostic Usefulness: Great: FRG, SWI, USA
Moderate: SWE, FRG

Procedure: The patient is prone. The patient's pelvis is stabilized with a belt. The arm opposite to the side of treatment hangs freely from the examination table. The ipsilateral leg (non-treatment side) is flexed to a maximum, and the patient's sole of the foot rests on the floor. The lumbar spine is rotated away from the treatment side (Fig. 262). The knee on the opposite side (treatment side) rests on over a pillow. Alternatively, the end of the examination table can be raised so as to introduce maximal tension in the muscle (which can also be achieved by sidebending the lumbar spine). To examine the iliopsoas muscle the thigh is externally rotated and extended (Fig. 263).

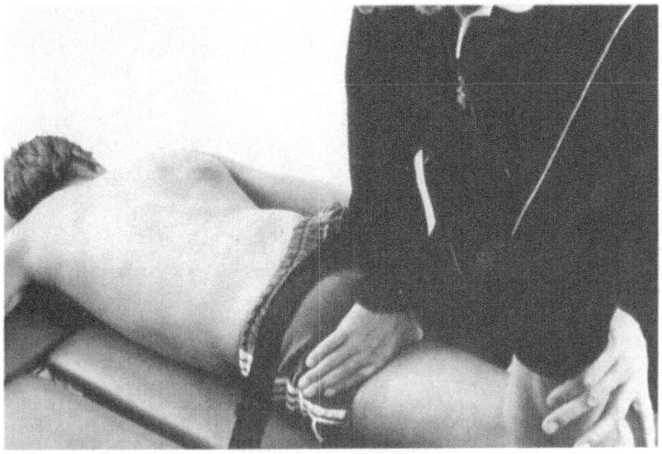

Fig. 262

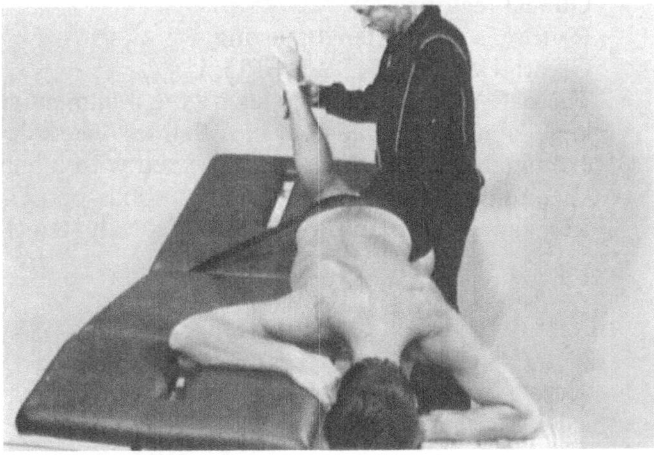

Fig. 263

Spinal Area: Hip region
Type of Examination: Length testing of the tensor fasciae latae
Diagnostic Usefulness: Great: USA, FRG, SWI, SWE
Moderate: I
Procedure: The patient is in the lateral recumbant position. Evaluated is the leg close to the examination table (in this case the inferior leg). The leg distal to the examination table (superior) is flexed approximately 90° in the hip and knee joints (a pillow is placed under the superior knee joint). The pelvis is stabilized with a belt. The leg is tested by introducing extension and external rotation (Fig. 264).

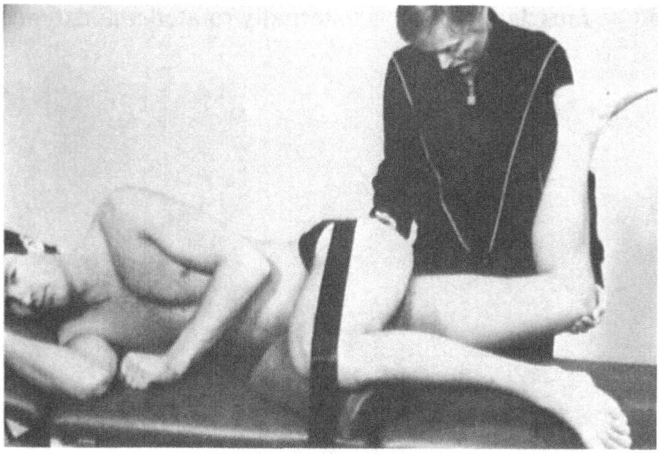

Fig. 264

Spinal Area: Gluteal region
Type of Examination: Piriformis muscle length testing
Diagnostic Usefulness: Great: USA, SWE, SWI, FRG, I
Procedure: The patient is supine, The leg on the treatment side is flexed at the hip and knee joint and placed over the other leg. The sole of the foot rests flat on the examination table. The pelvis is fixed with a belt. The operator pushes the knee in a medial direction along an axis perpendicular to the body's axis. Resistance and pain provocation are evaluated (Fig. 265).

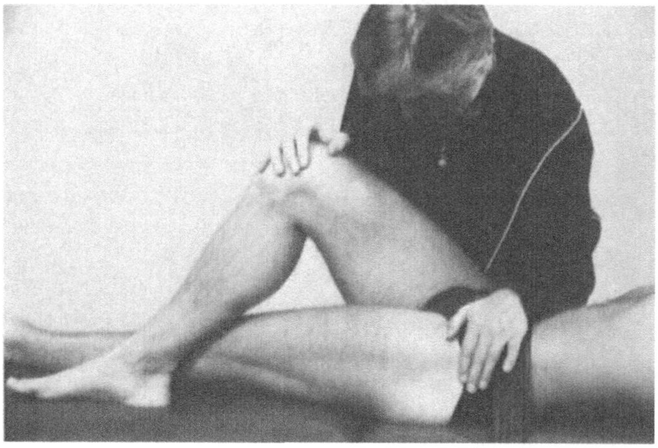

Fig. 265

6.3 Treatment

6.3.1 Treatment Procedures – General Comments

1. Passive Mobilization
2. Muscle Energy Technique
   The muscle energy technique (MET) is defined as the use of the patient's own muscle force to change the active and passive motion barrier and to improve muscle balance related to the dysfunctional area. The physiological mechanism underlying this technique is that of post-isometric relaxation.
3. Adjunct Procedures
   - Respiratory excursion
   - Eye movements which may reflexly influence the facilitation-inhibition-mechanism of the paraspinal muscles
4. Muscle Stretch Techniques
   - The muscle in question is monitored by the operator introducing tension in that muscle by positioning until the shortening can be felt both by the operator and the patient (position of unease).
   - Optimal isometric contraction of the shortened muscle
   - Muscle stretch should occur under the proper amount of force and time which in turn depends of the individual case.
   - Of importance for muscle stretch technique are the following muscles in the lumbo-sacral region: longissimus lumborum muscle, iliospinalis lumborum muscle, iliopsoas muscle, tensor fasciae latae muscle, adductor muscles, and hamstrings muscles

   Comparing the muscle stretch technique with the muscle energy technique (utilized by the American osteopathic physicians) their similarities became apparent: both utilize the neurophysiological mechanism of post-isometric relaxation.
5. Massage Techniques
   - Lateral stretch technique
   - Longitudinal stretching of the muscles. Pressure massage on tender origin- and insertion-tendinoses (which may be explained on the basis of the stimulation of type II mechanoreceptors resulting in the presynaptic inhibition of the nociceptive transmission in the region of the dorsal horn of the spinal cord)
6. Manipulation (Mobilization With Impulse-Thrust Techniques)
   With the patient in the lateral recumbant position, the pathological barrier of a spinal segment is engaged, and light traction is applied to the lumbar spine along the body's longitudinal axis. The thrusting force (impulse) is applied against the pathological barrier. This type of treatment should only be carried out by a physician who has experience in this form of treatment. In this maneuver, the spine proximal and distal to the spinal segment that is treated should be completely fixed (engaged). In the Swiss school, the direction of treatment is according to the segmental zone of irritation, with the impulse directed towards the zone of irritation.

6.3.2 Soft Tissue Treatment

Type of Treatment: Massage
Goal: Massage of the deep muscle layers in the lumbar region
Technique: Massage
Therapeutic Usefulness: Great: FRG
Moderate: SWI, USA, SWE
Little: I
Procedure: The patient is prone. Deep pressure massage is applied through the thumbs along the fiber direction of the deep muscle layers (Fig. 266).
Remarks: This is one aspect of the classical massage.

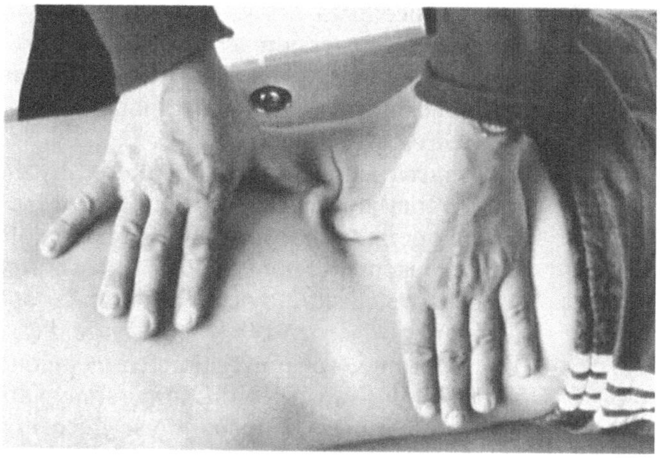

Fig. 266

6.3.3 Mobilization Without Impulse (No Thrust)

Type of Treatment: Mobilization without impulse (thrust)
Goal: Improvement of rotation and extension
Technique: Rotation mobilization
Therapeutic Usefulness: Great: I, FRG
Little: USA, SWI, SWE
Procedure: The patient is in the lateral recumbant position and the vertebral column is rotated and flexed. In this example, the operator guides his right arm under the patient's shoulder placing the hand close to the spinous process on the left side thus preventing its further movement while the opposite (left) hand and forearm rotate the pelvis to the left (Fig. 267).

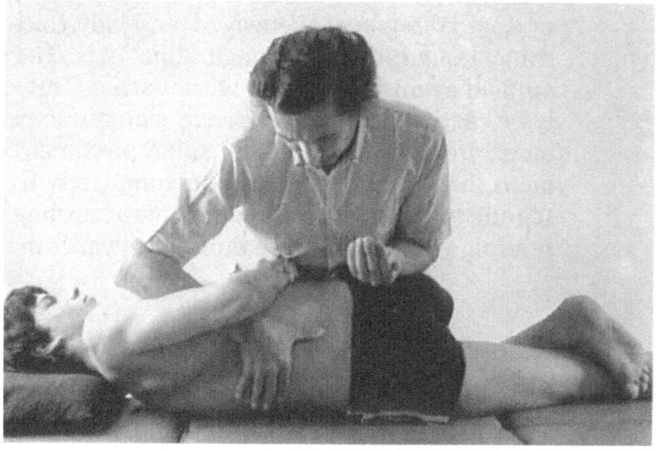

Fig. 267

Type of Treatment: Mobilization utilizing direct muscle contraction
Goal: Correction of an inferior pubic bone
Technique: Mobilization
Therapeutic Usefulness: Great: USA (osteopathic physicians), FRG
Little: SWE, USA, SWI
None: I
Procedure: The patient is supine with both hip and knee flexed (the right leg, for instance). The operator's left hand pushes on the ischial tuberocity towards the symphysis. Isometric extension of the right knee and hip is directed against a counterforce provided by the operator's right shoulder (Fig. 268).

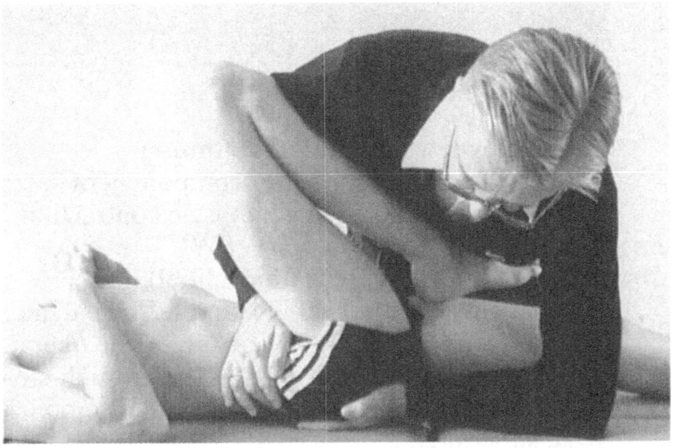

Fig. 268

Type of Treatment: Mobilization utilizing direct muscle contraction
Goal: Correction of a posterior sacrum
Treatment: Mobilization
Therapeutic Usefulness: Great: USA (osteopathic schools), FRG
Moderate: USA
Little: SWE, SWI, I
Procedure: The patient is in the lateral recumbent position and with rotation and extension movements introduced in the lumbar spine. In the example, the extended right leg is isometrically abducted against a counterforce (Fig. 269). The operator's right index finger monitors movement of the sacrum (Fig. 270).

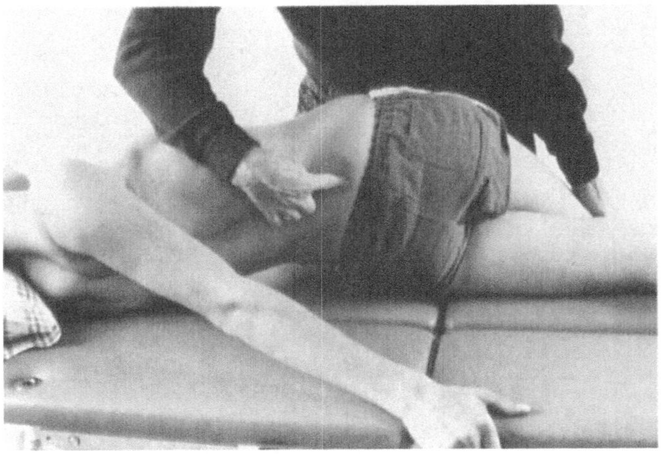

Fig. 269

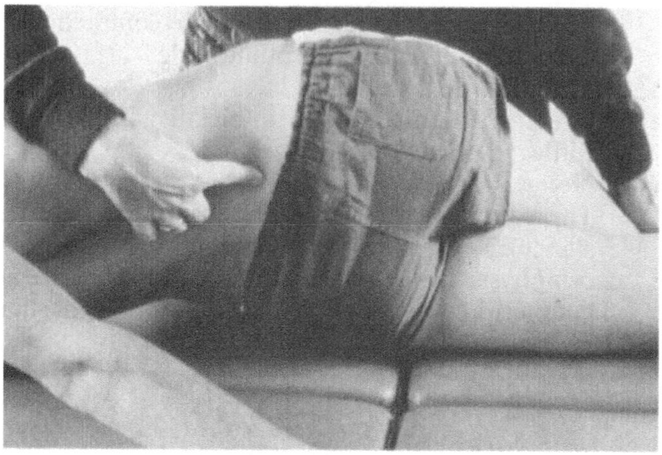

Fig. 270

Type of Treatment: Mobilization without impulse (thrust)

Goal: Improvement of the superior component of sacroiliac joint nutation

Technique: Mobilization utilizing direct muscle contraction

Therapeutic Usefulness: Moderate: USA, FRG, SWE, SWI
None: USA (osteopathic school), I

Procedure: The patient is prone. In this example, the patient's right anterior iliac spine is placed against the examination table. The operator's right hand palpates the sacro-tuberous ligament (Fig. 271). Through slow, deep exhalation and inhalation effort the right sacroiliac joint is mobilized. The right ilium is mobilized superiorly.

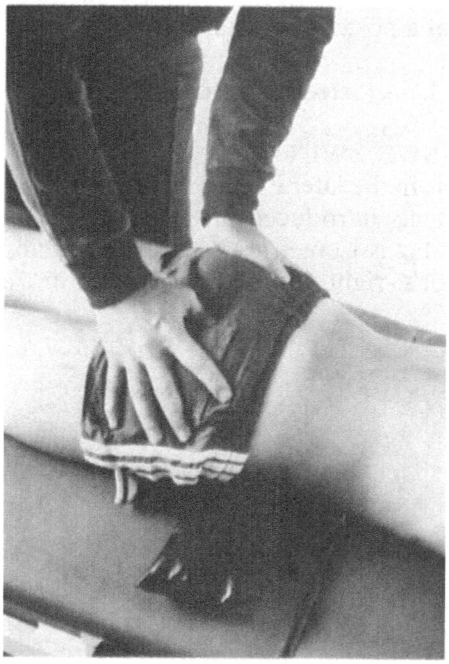

Fig. 271

Type of Treatment: Mobilization utilizing direction muscle contraction
Goal: Improvement of left sidebending and rotation
Treatment: Rotation and flexion mobilization
Therapeutic Usefulness: Great: USA (osteopathic school), FRG
Moderate: USA, SWI, SWE
Little: I

Procedure: The patient is in the lateral recumbant position. Rotation is introduced in the vertebral column such that the shoulder girdle comes to rest flat on the examination table. The hip and knees are flexed, while the spinous processes (i.e., L4–L5) are monitored by the operator's right hand. The operator's left hand provides a counterforce to the patient's right leg, which resists the patient's isometric internal rotation and external rotation effort in the right and in the left hip respectively (Fig. 272).

Remarks: Contracting the erector spinae muscles and the quadratus lumborum muscle has a mobilizing effect in the lumbar spinal segments. Postisometric relaxation of these muscles following isometric contraction will further enhance the therapeutic effect.

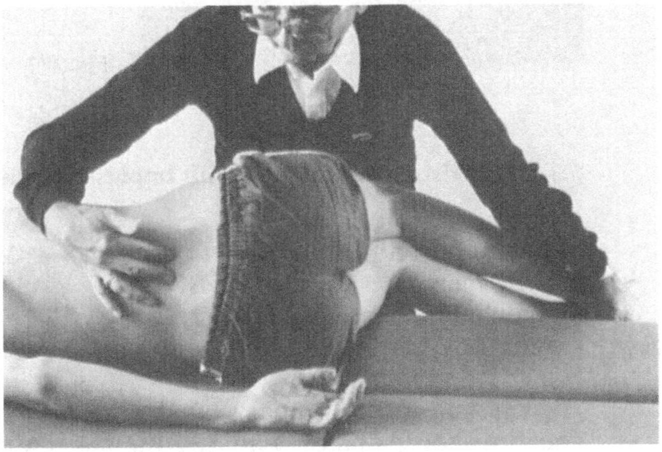

Fig. 272

Type of Treatment: Functional, indirect ease and bind technique
Goal: Improvement of flexion, sidebending and rotation in the lumbar spine
Technique: Functional, indirect ease and bind technique
Therapeutic Usefulness: Great: USA (osteopathic school), FRG
Little: SWI, SWE, USA, I

Procedure: The patient is sitting with the legs abducted. The operator palpates and monitors the interspinous spaces (i.e., L4–L5). In this example, the patient while extended is rotated to the right by the operator's left hand (Fig. 274). The exhalation and inhalation effort is utilized.

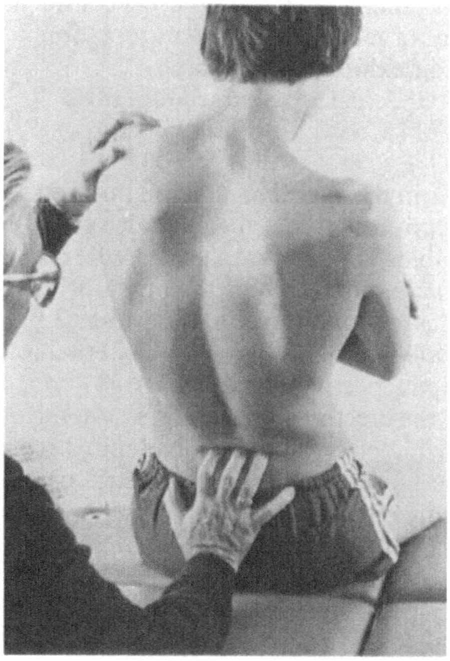

Fig. 273

6.3.4 Mobilizing Techniques With Impulse (Thrust)

Type of Treatment: Mobilization with impulse
Goal: Improvement of extension (L5–S1)
Technique: Manipulation to improve flexion
Therapeutic Usefulness: Little: USA, SWE, FRG, SWI
None: I
Procedure: The kneeling patient supports his shoulder girdle on the examination table. The operator palpates with his thumbs the mamillary process at L5 (Fig. 274). The impulse applied to L5 is in an anterior direction. The operator introduces low amplitude, high velocity thrust by extending the elbows from their originally flexed position and immediately removing the hands after the thrusting force has been applied.

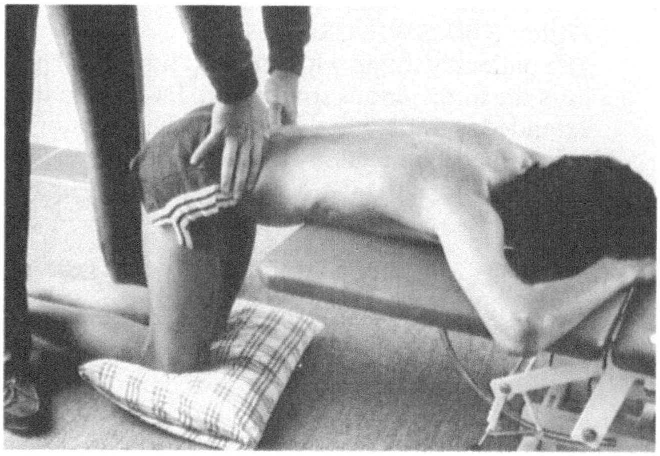

Fig. 274

Type of Treatment: Mobilization with impulse
Goal: Improvement of extension, sidebending and rotation.
Technique: Manipulation for extension, sidebending, rotation
Therapeutic Usefulness: Great: USA
Little: SWE, FRG
None: I
Procedure: The patient is sitting. In this example, the patient's lumbar spine is extended, sidebent and rotated to the right. The impulse is effected through the operator's left thumb upon the right side of the spinous process of L4 (Fig. 275).

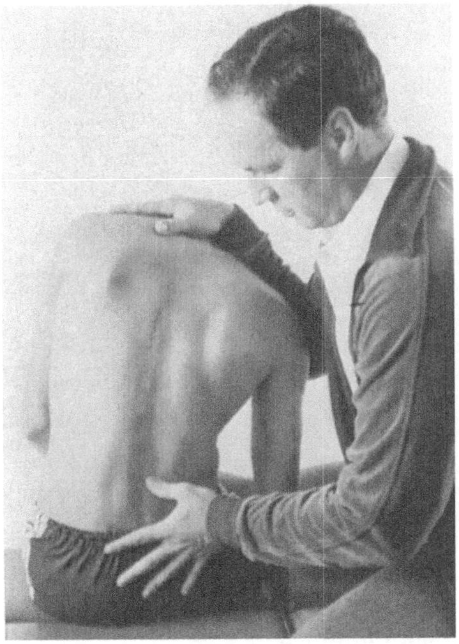

Fig. 275

Type of Treatment: Mobilization with impulse
Goal: Improvement of flexion, sidebending and rotation in the lumbar spine
Technique: Rotation manipulation
Therapeutic Usefulness: Great: FRG, USA (osteopathic school)
Moderate: I, SWE, SWI
None: USA
Procedure: In this example, the patient is in the left lateral recumbant position. Rotation and flexion are introduced to engage the barriers of the vertebral column (Fig. 276). With his right hand, the operator stabilizes the spinous process of L4 and introduces the impulse in the direction of right rotation while with the left hand he stabilizes and thrusts through the spinous process of L5 following the left rotation direction (Fig. 277).

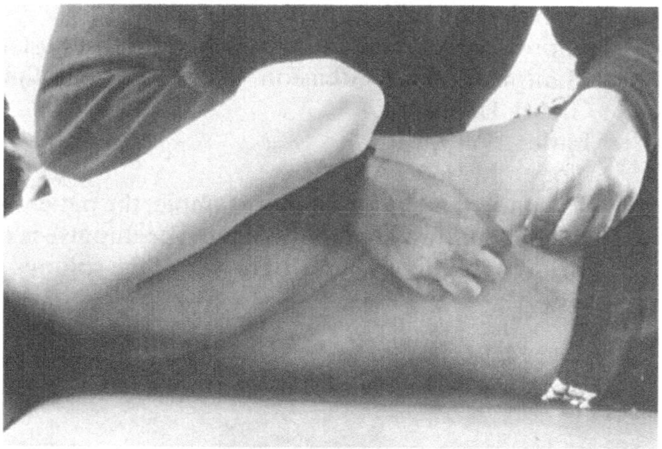

Fig. 276

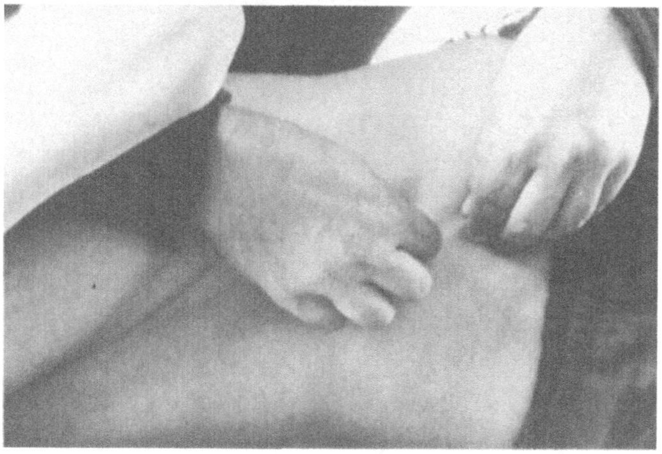

Fig. 277

Type of Treatment: Mobilization with impulse
Goal: Improvement of extension, sidebending and rotation in the lumbar spine
Technique: Rotation manipulation
Therapeutic Usefulness: Great: I
Moderate: USA
Little: USA (osteopathic school), FRG, SWE, SWI
Procedure: The patient is sitting on the examination table with his legs apart. Flexion is introduced so as to bring the vertebral column to its barrier, and the rotation and sidebending to the right are introduced (as in this example). With his left pisiform bone the operator palpates the patient's left transverse process of L4. The impulse follows right rotation and flexion (Fig. 278).

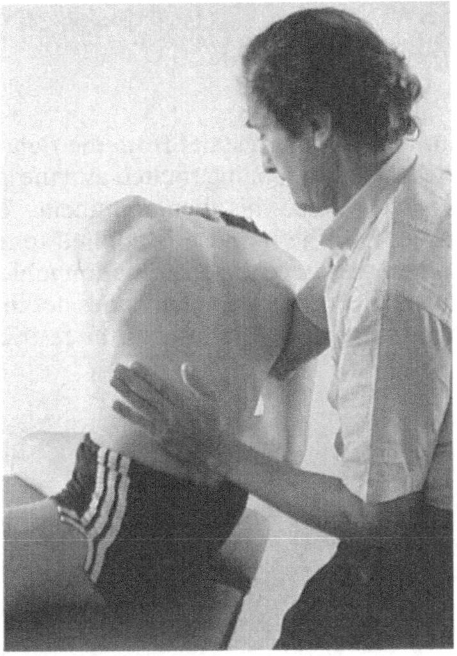

Fig. 278

Type of Treatment: Mobilization with impulse
Goal: Improvement of flexion, sidebending and rotation in the L5–S1 spinal segment
Technique: Rotation and extension manipulation
Therapeutic Usefulness: Great: I
Little: USA, FRG, SWE, SWI
Procedure: The patient's pelvis is stabilized with a belt. In this example, the supine patient is rotated so that his right arm will rest over the operator's right shoulder. The impulse is directed towards the spinous process of L5 with the operator's left hand following right rotation (Fig. 279). Simultaneous extension motion at the lumbar spine is effected by the operator lifting his right shoulder against the patient.

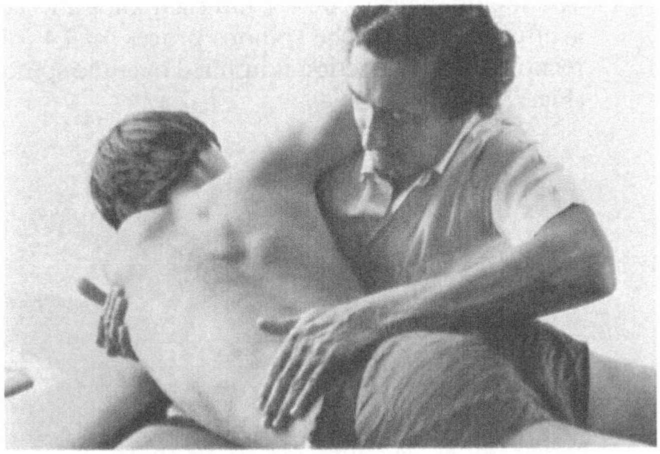

Fig. 279

Type of Treatment: Mobilization with impulse
Goal: Mobilization of the lumbar spine
Technique: Rotation manipulation

Therapeutic Usefulness: Great: SWI
Moderate: FRG
Little: I, SWE
None: USA

Procedure: In this example, the patient starts from the right lateral recumbant position with the vertebral column being rotated and the shoulder and left knee stabilized. The operator places his thenar eminence over the left side of the spinous process of L4. The impulse is applied to the spinous process follows left rotation in direction of the examination table (Fig. 280).

Remarks: This manipulative procedure actually does not improve motion, since the direction of manipulation is not towards the restricted barrier.

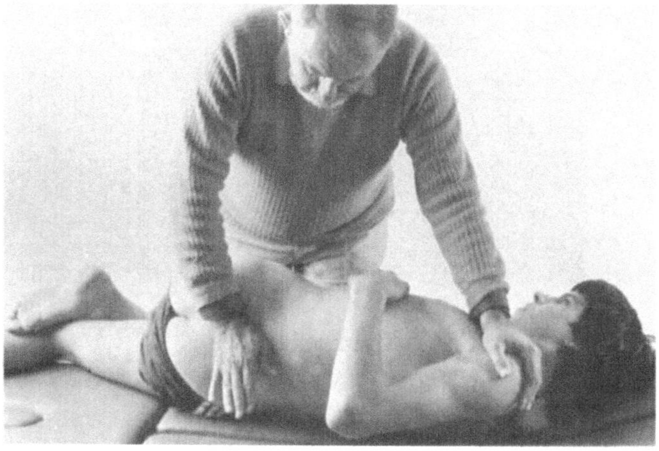

Fig. 280

Type of Treatment: Mobilization with impulse (thrust)
Goal: Improvement of the lumbar spine rotation
Technique: Rotation manipulation
Therapeutic Usefulness: Great: SWI, FRG
Moderate: SWE
Little: USA, I

Procedure: The patient is in the sidelying position with the vertebral column rotated. The shoulder girdle, pelvis and right knee are stabilized. The thrusting force is effected through the spinous process at L4 following the left rotation direction. Inferior traction is applied over the spinous process of L4 and pelvis (Fig. 281).

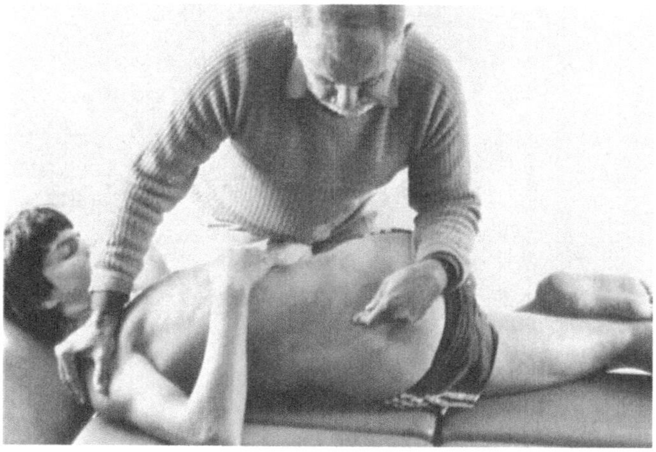

Fig. 281

Type of Treatment: Mobilization with impulse
Goal: Improvement of flexion and rotation in the lumbar spine
Technique: Rotation manipulation
Therapeutic Usefulness: Great: I, FRG
Little: USA, SWI, SWE
Procedure: The patient is in the sidelying position with the spine rotated and the lumbar spine extended. In this example, the operator's right arm is placed under the patient's right shoulder, and his right thumb contacts the right side of the spinous process of L4 (Fig. 282). The left forearm is placed over the patient's pelvis, and a rotatory impulse is applied through the right hand and the right elbow following the right rotation. A simultaneous impulse is applied to the pelvis following the left rotation direction.

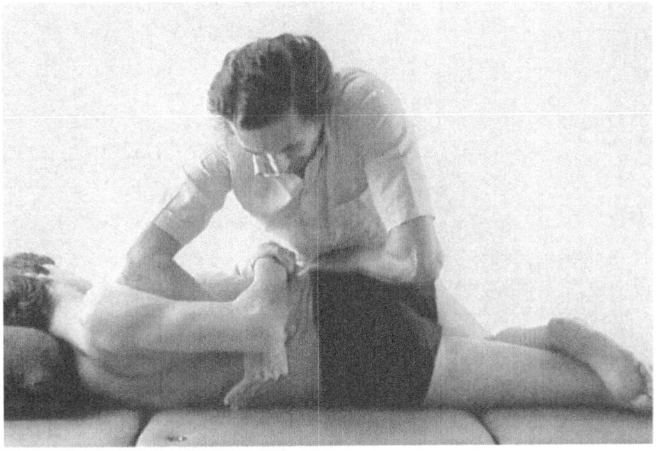

Fig. 282

Type of Treatment: Mobilization with impulse
Goal: Improvement of anterior nutation mobility in the sacroiliac joint
Technique: Sacroiliac joint manipulation
Therapeutic Usefulness: Great: USA
Moderate: USA (osteopathic physicians)
Little: SWI, SWE, FRG
Procedure: The patient is in the lateral recumbant position. The vertebral column is brought to its barrier through rotation. The operator introduces with his left hand an anteriorly directed impulse on the right ischial tuberosity (Fig. 283).

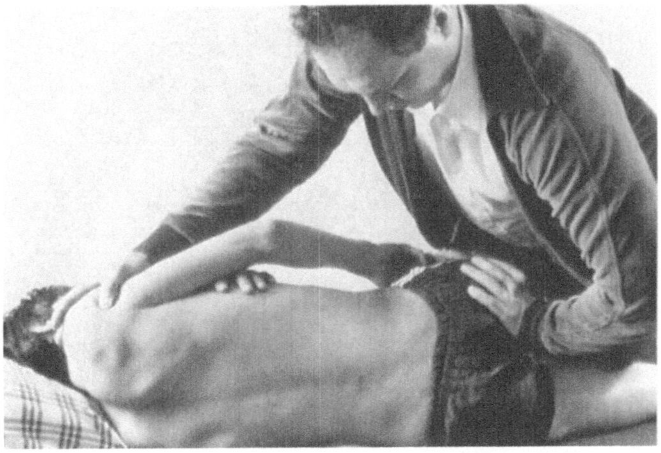

Fig. 283

Type of Treatment: Mobilization with impulse
Goal: Improvement of the nutation motion in the sacroiliac joint as well as improvement of soft tissues in the right sacroiliac joint.
Technique: Sacroiliac joint manipulation
Therapeutic Usefulness: Great: SWI
Moderate: FRG, USA, SWE
None: USA, I
Procedure: The patient is prone. As demonstrated in this example, the operator's left hand palpates with the ulnar border the patient's right sacrum. The other hand palpates the patient's right iliac crest. The impulse is in an anterior direction and is applied to the right sacrum with simultaneous lateral motion over the ilium (Fig. 284).

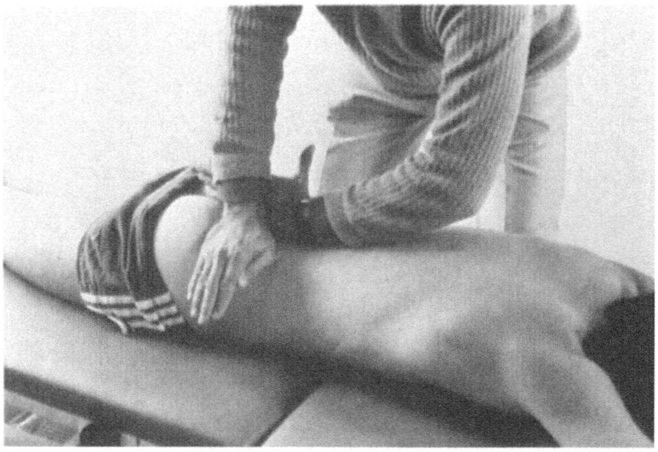

Fig. 284

Type of Treatment: Mobilization with impulse
Goal: Nutation improvement at the sacroiliac joint
Technique: Sacroiliac joint manipulation
Therapeutic usefulness: Great: SWI
Moderate: SWE, USA, FRG
None: I
Procedure: In this example, the patient is in the right sidelying position, and left rotation in the vertebral column is introduced. The impulse following a left rotation direction is directed towards the right sacrum by the pisiform bone and the fifth metacarpal of the operator's right hand (Fig. 285).

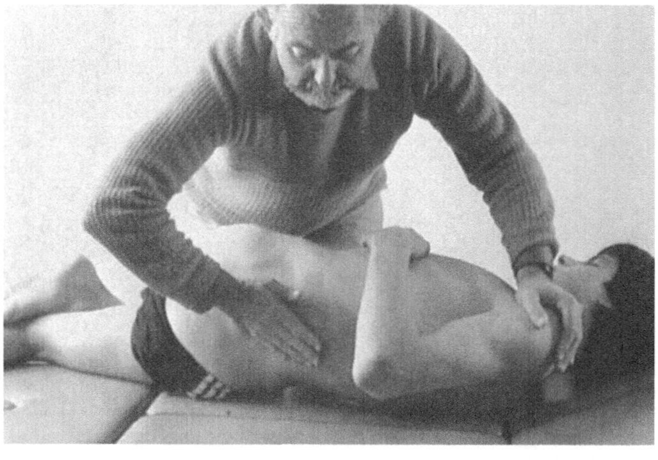

Fig. 285

Type of Treatment: Mobilization with impulse
Goal: Improvement of nutation motion in the right sacroiliac joint
Technique: Sacroiliac joint manipulation
Therapeutic Usefulness: Great: SWI
Moderate: USA, SWE, FRG
None: I
Procedure: As presented in this example, the patient is in the left lateral position with the vertebral column rotated to the right. The shoulder girdle is stabilized. The hand is placed flat over the right ilium. The impulse is to the left following the direction of pelvis rotation (Fig. 286).

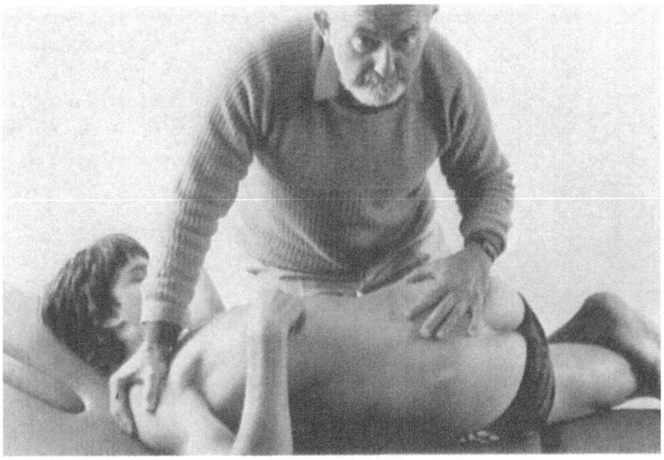

Fig. 286

6.3.5 Muscle Rehabilitation

Type of Treatment: Muscle stretching without utilization of postisometric relaxation
Goal: Stretching of the shortened erector spinae muscles in the lumbar region
Technique: Muscle stretch technique
Therapeutic Usefulness: Great: FRG
Moderate: USA, SWE, SWI
Little: I
Procedure: The patient is prone, and the erector spinae muscles in the lumbar region (i. e., left side) are pushed laterally to the left as well as anteriorly with the operator's hand (Fig. 287).

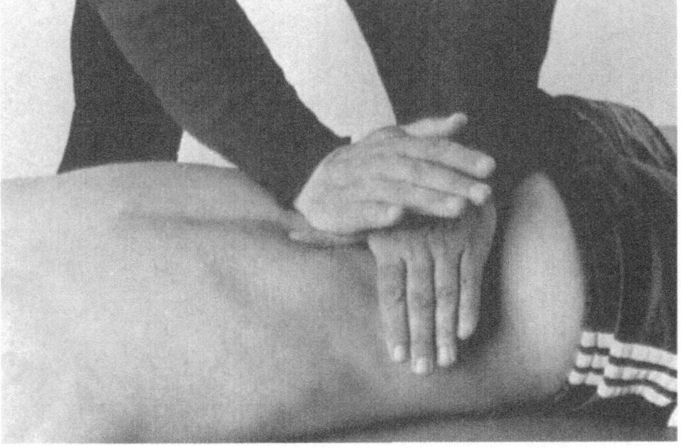

Fig. 287

Type of Treatment: Muscle stretching without utilization of post-isometric relaxation
Goal: Stretching of the erector spinae muscles in the lumbar region
Technique: Muscle stretch technique
Therapeutic Usefulness: Great: FRG
Moderate: USA, I, SWI, SWE
Procedure: The patient is in the lateral recumbant position (i.e., left) with the lumbar spine somewhat extended. With the fingers of both hands the operator palpates the right lumbar erector spinae muscles and performs lateral stretching. This stretching force is further enhanced by the operator leaning on the patient's shoulder girdle and pelvis (Fig. 288).

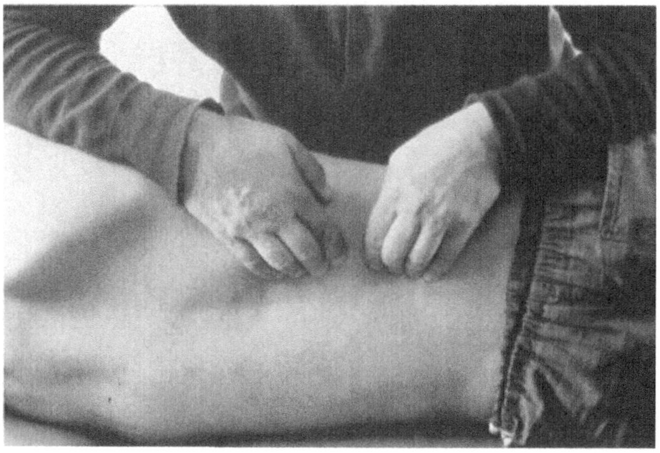

Fig. 288

Treatment: Muscle stretching utilizing post-isometric relaxation
Goal: Stretching of the hamstring muscles
Therapeutic Usefulness: Great: SWE, FRG, SWI, USA
Little: I
Procedure: The patient is supine and his right hip and knee are flexed while the thigh is stabilized with a belt. The ipsilateral foot is placed against the operator's right shoulder. The patient's left thigh is further stabilized with the operator's right hand (Fig. 289). With resistance against the operator's right shoulder isometric knee flexion is introduced. During post-isometric relaxation (Fig. 290), the hamstring muscles are stretched in a stepwise manner by extending the knee joint.

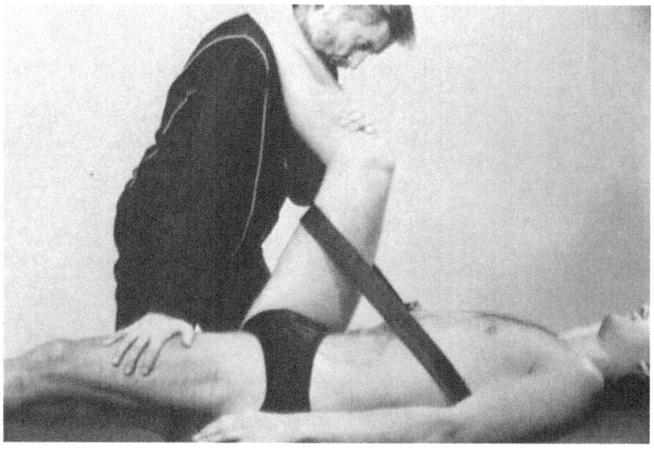

Fig. 289

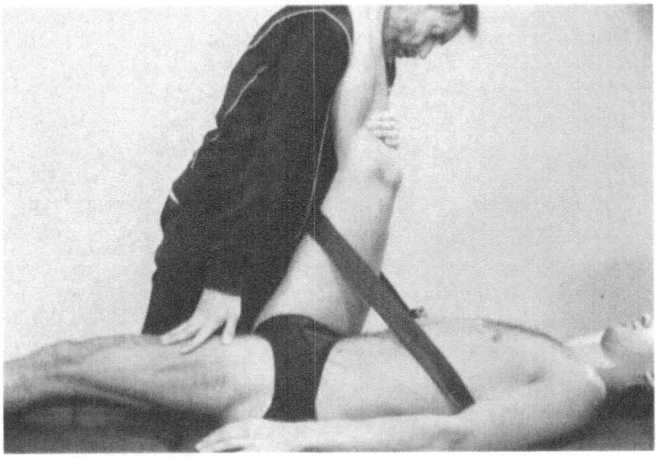

Fig. 290

Type of Treatment: Muscle stretching utilizing post-isometric relaxation

Goal: Stretching of the shortened iliopsoas muscle

Technique: Muscle stretch technique

Therapeutic Usefulness: Great: SWE, USA (osteopathic school), SWI, FRG
Moderate: USA
Little: I

Procedure: The patient is prone. In this example, the patient's left leg, which rests on the floor, is flexed at both the knee and hip joints. The pelvis is stabilized with a belt. The right knee is then flexed 90°. The pelvis is stabilized by the operator's left hand. With the left leg and hip fixed the operator controls the patient's pelvis and lumbar spine positions. The right hand reaches around the patient's right knee while the patient's right lower leg and foot are being placed against the operator's right shoulder (Fig. 291).
Isometric flexion at the right hip joint is then effected against the table. During the postisometric relaxation phase the end of the table is lifted introducing passive flexion at the right hip joint. Moving his shoulder simultaneously the operator increases internal rotation in the right hip joint (Fig. 292).

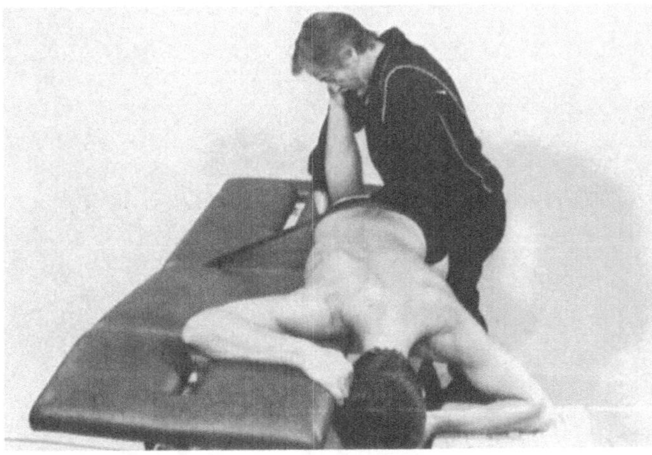

Fig. 291

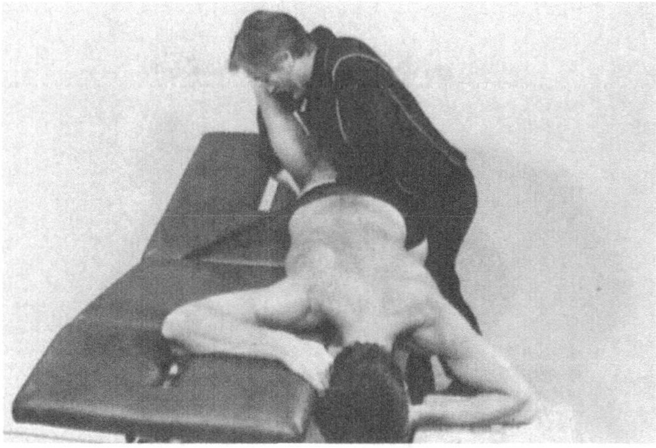

Fig. 292

Type of Treatment: Muscle stretch technique utilizing post-isometric relaxation
Goal: Stretching of the shortened piriformis muscle
Technique: Muscle stretch technique
Therapeutic Usefulness: Great: SWI, USA, FRG
Moderate: SWE, I

Procedure: The patient is supine with the right hip flexed 60° and the right knee flexed also. The left hip is then adducted as to have the left foot margin touch the right lower leg. The patient's pelvis is stabilized by the operator's left arm and the use of a belt. Resistence is also provided to the right knee joint (Fig. 293). Isometric abduction and external rotation motions are then effected. During the post-isometric relaxation phase the piriformis muscle is stretched by further adduction in the right hip joint (Fig. 294).

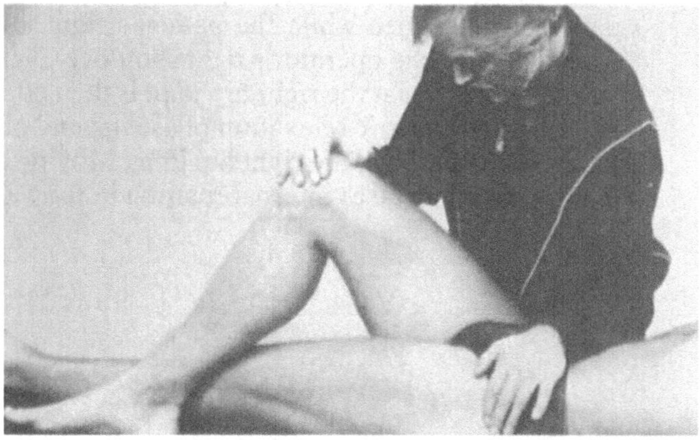

Fig. 293

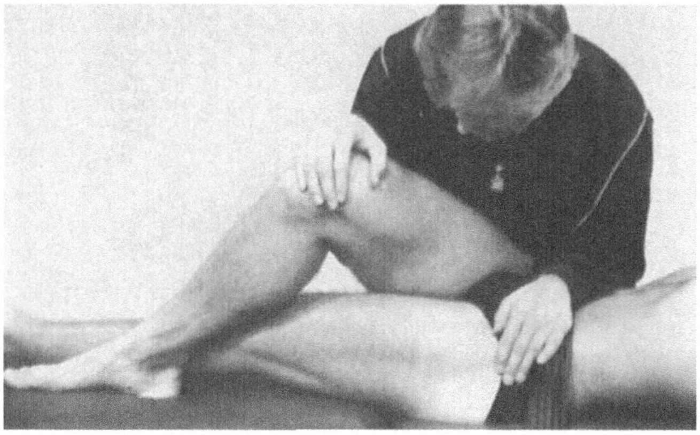

Fig. 294

Type of Treatment: Muscle stretching utilizing post-isometric relaxation
Goal: Stretching of the tensor fasciae latae muscle
Technique: Muscle stretch technique
Therapeutic Usefulness: Great: SWE, SWI, USA (osteopathic school), FRG
Moderate: USA
Little: I

Procedure: The patient in this example is in the right lateral recumbant position. The left knee and hip are flexed. By stabilizing the patient's pelvis with a belt and pillow and the patient's left thigh with the right hand, the operator fixes the sacrum and the ilium.

With the left hand the operator holds the patient's right knee and places the patient's right foot against his left shoulder (Fig. 295).

Isometric contraction is then effected against resistance at the right knee joint. During the post-isometric relaxation phase there is stepwise extension, adduction, and external rotation in the right hip joint (Fig. 296).

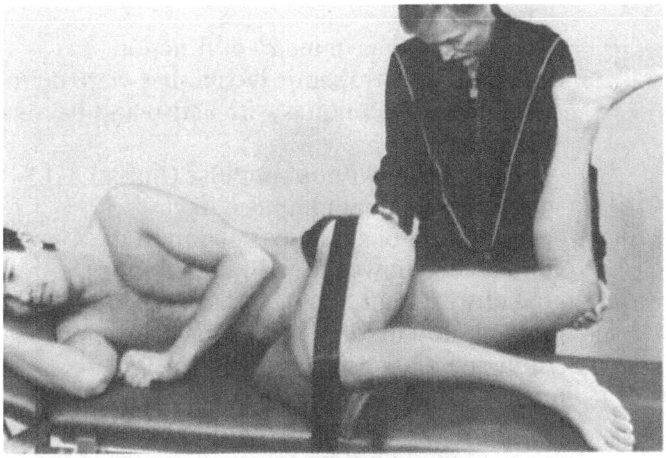

Fig. 295

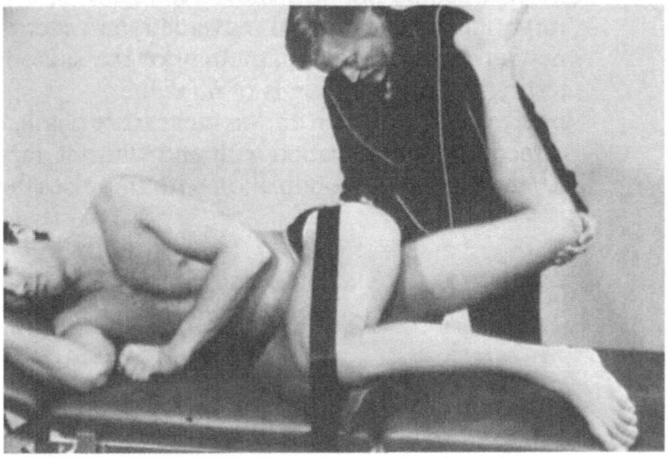

Fig. 296

6.4 Summary

After extensive discussions the major goal of manual medicine was formulated as follows:
To achieve maximum painfree range of motion in static and dynamic balance of the musculo-skeletal system.

The group defined basic concepts in three areas:

1. Basic biomechanic principles
   - lumbar mobility
   - sacral movement in walking
   - sacral movement in forward bending and sidebending
   - innominate movement and movement of symphysis pubis.
2. Diagnostic Criteria and Techniques
   - soft tissue techniques
   - pain and pain provocation
   - mobility
   - balance and asymmetry of function
3. Principles of therapeutic techniques were defined as:
   - soft tissue techniques with active and passive stretching of muscles and tissues
   - mobilization without impulse (thrust)
   - mobilization with impulse (thrust)
   - restoration of somatic function in the musculoskeletal system

Major agreement was found in relation to:
- goal of treatment
- gross motion in multi-segmental movement
- soft tissue diagnosis
- muscle length and muscle strength testing
- mobilization with and without impulse (thrust) technique procedures

Agreement could not be achieved in regard to:
- importance of segmental movement and sacroiliac movement; Italy does neither recognize any pathology of the sacroiliac joint, and it finds that testing or manipulation is of no value.
- interpretation of pain and tissue texture changes in soft tissues
- direction of mobilization with and without impulse (thrust)
- levers applied in mobilization with impulse (thrust)

GPSR Compliance

The European Union's (EU) General Product Safety Regulation (GPSR) is a set of rules that requires consumer products to be safe and our obligations to ensure this.

If you have any concerns about our products, you can contact us on ProductSafety@springernature.com

In case Publisher is established outside the EU, the EU authorized representative is:

Springer Nature Customer Service Center GmbH
Europaplatz 3
69115 Heidelberg, Germany

Batch number: 10615099

Printed by Printforce, the Netherlands